Food Allergies

Food Allergies

*The Complete Guide to Understanding
and Relieving Your Food Allergies*

William E. Walsh, M.D., F.A.C.A

John Wiley & Sons, Inc.
New York ◊ Chichester ◊ Weinheim ◊ Brisbane ◊ Singapore ◊ Toronto

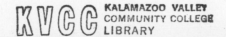

The information contained in this book is not intended to serve as a replacement for professional medical advice. Any use of the information in this book is at the reader's discretion. The author and the publisher specifically disclaim any and all liability arising directly or indirectly from the use or application of any information contained in this book. A health care professional should be consulted regarding your specific situation.

ISBN 0-471-38268-X

Printed in the United States of America

10 9 8 7 6 5 4 3 2 1

CONTENTS

ACKNOWLEDGMENTS

This book and the diet it describes would not exist without the help of many contributors. I am honored to acknowledge their help and to thank those whose generous assistance was so essential.

Much of the dietary advice contained in this book is new and surprising and was originally discovered, not by me, but by patients observant enough to recognize the foods and beverages responsible for their illnesses. These novel aspects of the diet became permanent additions when other patients found they were important in controlling their symptoms. To those patients whose insights shaped the diet and to those patients who followed the diet and confirmed its value, I extend a heartfelt thank you. I would never have the chance to describe the diet without your counsel and guidance.

Just as the help of my patients was essential in developing this diet, so, too, was the assistance of the registered nurses who work with me. Each has specialized for many years in the care of the allergic patient. My nurses and I approach the treatment of our allergic patients as a team, from initial evaluation and diagnosis through follow-up care. I express my gratitude to the nurses who work with me now and those who helped in the past: Arleen, Betty, Caryl, Connie, Corinne, Elaine, Jan, Kristie, Nikki, Peggy, and Shirley.

To my patients' pediatricians, family physicians, internists, physicians' assistants, nurse practitioners, chiropractors, and other medical care professionals, my heartfelt thanks. These dedicated men and women comfort my patients when they are sad, care for them when they are ill, and bring the benefits of modern medicine to their bedsides. Without them my practice would not be possible.

I am also grateful for the fine work and cooperation of Felicia Busch. Her expertise in the food sciences considerably enhances the value of this book for the food-sensitive person, and this expertise is readily apparent on examination of her practical advice.

Many others have contributed to the diet and the book, including Barbara Field and Martha King, whose skills with writing helped make sense of many murky passages. To all of you, my deepest thanks.

NOTE ABOUT
CASE HISTORIES

The case histories described in this book are representative of many conversations with patients who have similar illnesses and food allergies. They are included to help the reader understand food allergy and its treatment. Although the essence of each case history is preserved, the names, occupations, and certain facts have been changed to prevent recognition of the patients, to protect their privacy, and to better illustrate the ideas presented here.

PREFACE

When we go on a journey, we expect to complete it safely and at our destination. Yet that doesn't always happen. Think of the poor passengers on the *Titanic*, who paid their money to enjoy the maiden voyage of this luxurious ocean liner, content in the knowledge that the ship could not sink. Unfortunately, this bold claim made no impression on the iceberg that brought their voyage to disaster.

Fortunately, most of the time our journeys end safely and we reach our destination, usually with the help of a few key people. For instance, if you are traveling to Germany, you might first visit a travel agent, an expert in trip planning. To get to the airport, you call a cab; the driver is an expert in city transportation. You board a plane whose pilot is an expert in flying. You stay in a hotel staffed by experts in lodging. Your trip goes smoothly because competent experts handle each step.

A book is like a journey for your mind. You read it because you have a destination or a goal you want to reach; when you finish, you hope to have reached this goal. If the book is a detective story or a science fiction novel, you want excitement and entertainment; from a biography or a wildlife novel, you desire knowledge and adventure. From a medical book, you hope to gain the most precious knowledge of all, a way to improve your health.

That is the purpose of this book. I hope that when you complete your journey through its pages with me, you gain knowledge that helps you ease your pain and discomfort. And just as you have every right to question the qualifications of the people who help you on your make-believe trip to Germany, so you have every right to question my qualifications, since I am your travel guide, cabbie, and pilot on this trip. Let me give them to you.

I am a medical doctor with the same M.D. degree as a pediatrician, family doctor, or internist. After completing medical school, I served two years in the U.S. Air Force, where I had the opportunity to care for an allergy clinic. The field of allergy fascinated me, and I thought that I would be happy spending my life treating people with allergy problems

As I think back to those days, I find that my decision to be an allergist was right. I enjoy helping people who suffer from allergy.

When I originally decided to be an allergist, I also decided that the field is so complicated that I needed further training. I gained this training at the Mayo Clinic, where I spent four hardworking but enjoyable years. The clinic, through its expert teaching staff and diverse patient load, offers the allergist-in-training magnificent opportunities to study the many areas he or she is responsible for when treating people, areas such as allergic dermatology, allergic chest disease, and allergic gastrointestinal disease. I also learned how pollen, dust, and mold affect patients with allergy. Daily, I use this training to help me understand this demanding field.

After completing my training at the Mayo Clinic, I moved to St. Paul, Minnesota, in 1970, where I started my current allergy practice. Shortly afterward, I took and passed an examination certifying me as a specialist in allergy. The certificate is from the American Board of Allergy and Immunology and is recognized by the American Board of Pediatrics and the American Board of Internal Medicine.

The American Board of Allergy and Immunology sponsors active programs to keep allergists up to date, including providing the opportunity to retake allergy board examinations at intervals, a process called voluntary recertification. To ensure that my knowledge remained current, I have repeated the recertification exam and on each occasion earned my recertification diploma.

I have described my credentials to assure you that I wrote this book as a qualified allergy specialist who stays current with modern scientific knowledge of allergic illness. Although my training and diplomas give this medical book credibility, they are only part of the reason this book exists. Equally important are several other factors.

One factor makes me uniquely qualified to write this book: I myself suffer from allergic reactions to foods; I share with my patients and with you, the reader, this allergy. Perhaps that's fortunate—in a way. If you are looking for an authority in food allergy, who would be more appropriate than a doctor whose personal experience includes suffering from this allergy?

Because of my own sensitivity, food allergy fascinates me; who wouldn't be fascinated by a medical illness if he or she were its victim? I know it steered me toward my specialty in the first place, and I remember how it happened.

I was walking to work on a lovely fall day in 1965, looking quite nice in my spiffy air force captain's uniform. However, my mind wasn't on enjoying the warm, green Nebraska scenery; instead I felt confused and uncertain as I considered the many specialized fields of medicine my M.D. degree unlocked. Which one was right for me?

Should it be family medicine, with the satisfaction of caring for all the illnesses of my patients, of treating the whole patient, of being the first doctor they call when they are ill? On the other hand, maybe I should enter obstetrics, for the joy of delivering healthy babies and treating the illnesses of women. Or perhaps I was suited for plastic surgery, for the pride of restoring a ravished face, or psychiatry, with its awesome potential for healing the human mind.

Then the obvious struck me, and I stopped and laughed. There I was, standing in a green and weedy field at the height of the fall ragweed pollen season, my eyes running like a crying baby's and my nose dripping like old plumbing with a leak, wheezing like a couch potato running a marathon. To add to my miseries, my armpits were itching from contact dermatitis to a deodorant I had used that morning. I said to myself, "Bill, whatever could you be other than an allergist?"

I have never regretted that decision, and as I pick up new allergies, they serve to reinforce and renew my interest in, and fascination for, the field of allergy. When foods began to trouble me, my attention to food allergy increased enormously, especially when articles in the allergy literature started questioning whether allergists paid enough attention to patients' complaints about food. I discovered I paid little attention, and I resolved to change.

Making resolutions is as easy as eating when hungry and drinking when thirsty. Keeping resolutions is as hard as growing food in a drought or finding water in a desert. However, I kept my resolve to study food allergy because of my own food reactions.

Unfortunately, I found that treating food allergy was uncommonly difficult. Why? Because my patients told me about symptoms that the allergy literature said did not happen. They told me about reactions to foods that allergists taught were harmless. As my patients' stories about their food allergies continued to contradict the allergy literature, I became more confused and more frustrated.

I knew I needed to learn more about food allergy, but I did not know where to turn to acquire this knowledge. I could either choose to accept my specialty's teachings about food allergy, or I could choose to believe my patients when they told me their weird-sounding stories of food reactions. I chose to believe my patients.

I'm glad I did. Over a period of years, their strange tales started to make sense. A pattern of food allergy emerged, and a dietary approach to healing was born. I wish I could say this diet sprang from my brilliant deductions, but that's not true. It arose from my patients' observations as they taught me the diet a little at a time.

I learned as they related their discoveries about the foods that aggravated their headaches, hives, and diarrhea. Each discovery lessened the confusion surrounding food allergy; each discovery added another important element to the diet.

This brings me to why I wrote *Food Allergies*. I wrote it for several reasons, but the first and most important reason involves my patients. I wrote it for them. I am so very proud of them. The poker game of life dealt them a miserable hand. They live a life full of headaches, stuffy noses, wheezing, skin itchiness and rashes, abdominal discomfort, achiness, tiredness, and other illnesses.

Many people suffering similar tribulations give up; they stop trying to conquer their illnesses. They accept their pain and misfortune, and they comfort themselves with self-pity to soothe their distress.

Not my patients. They persevered. Although many people—including some doctors—tried to discourage them from finding the reasons for their distress, they never stopped looking. The search brought them to my office and ultimately to the dietary changes that form such a large part of their treatment.

By their perseverance, they amply demonstrate their determination. They continue to advance, never quitting. They are heroic.

Through this book I want to better explain to you, the reader, how to find your own food allergies and to help guide you through the many dietary choices you must make each day. Many have told me the information I present in this book does just that—helps them gain this knowledge to better understand food allergy and why we suffer from it.

How many people in various walks of life suffer because they do not know that allergy causes pain and illness? Unfortunately, I believe the answer is many. I hope this book helps them. If it does—if people I will never meet gain relief from their food-caused illness—I will be pleased. Their health is a reward that gives me great delight.

CHAPTER 1

An Introduction to Food Allergy

We Begin Our Journey to Better Health

You are reading this book because you or a loved one are suffering. You suspect that foods may be part of the cause of this suffering, but you are not sure that the symptoms that plague you could arise from your diet. If they do, which foods must you avoid? I specialize in helping people who suffer from food allergy and, through this book, I will try to help you find the answers to these questions.

As to the first question—what symptoms can foods cause?—the answer is many. My food-sensitive patients suffer symptoms that you probably know are allergic, including hives, eczema, congestion, wheezing, and sneezing. Sometimes their symptoms are scary and dangerous, such as choking and fainting that may end in unconsciousness. They also suffer symptoms that you may not realize are caused by allergy, such as tiredness, poor concentration, headaches, stomach aches, diarrhea, numb areas of the body, and aching joints and muscles. If you suffer from these symptoms, I will tell you how they arise.

As we explore food allergy I will also answer the second question: Which foods cause these symptoms? By knowing which of your symptoms could be caused by foods and which foods to suspect, you can learn to live a life without pain and discomfort.

But you need more than lists of symptoms and foods to successfully treat yourself. You need to understand why food allergy exists. You should know principles of diagnosis and treatment so you can decide what actions you need to take. I will try to teach you this.

Understanding and treating food allergy are like building a house. The symptoms and suspect foods are the framing, walls, windows, and doors of the house. They need a firm foundation, or they will collapse. As you would start building a house by forming this foundation, we will begin our study of food allergy by examining general information about food allergy and some of the principles that should guide your thoughts and actions.

Once we establish this foundation, we will then look at the foods that cause allergic symptoms. Finally, we will put the roof on our study of food allergy by summarizing what we learned as we apply this knowledge to treating your food allergy.

Before going further, I should give you a word of caution to help you use this book wisely.

Don't Try to Make This Book Your Doctor

I wrote this book to tell you my methods of treating food allergy so you can apply them to your own life. I did not write it to tell you how to diagnose these illnesses without assistance. Diagnosing illness is the specialty of your primary care professional. Let him or her help you diagnose your illness.

In my allergy practice, I try to make sure each of my patients has a primary medical care professional who has already diagnosed allergy and excluded—as far as possible—nonallergic illness as the cause of my patients' symptoms. If you were my patient and we questioned the cause of your illness, I would send you to your primary doctor for diagnosis. Go to him or her now if there is any question about your diagnosis. If your doctor wants help in diagnosis, he or she may suggest you see a neurologist, dermatologist, or other specialist; if so, take this advice.

Maintain a Healthy Diet
While You Follow My Dietary Advice

Some of the foods and beverages I ask you to avoid add no value to a healthy diet. Other foods and beverages are championed by dietary experts who teach us they are a necessary part of a healthy diet (a number of dieticians are scandalized that we ask our patients to exclude them). Excluding these foods and beverages is not fatal to a healthy diet. There are plenty of healthy foods you can eat while you avoid the foods that cause you pain and discomfort.

In certain circumstances there is a danger you will slip into a nutritionally inadequate and therefore unhealthy diet. For instance, if you already follow a medically prescribed diet that excludes healthy foods, and you also try to exclude the foods and beverages that trouble my patients, your diet may be inadequate and your health threatened. The same threat could surface if you follow a diet not prescribed by a skilled primary care professional. If there is any chance that your diet will become inadequate and unhealthy, do not follow my diet until you consult your medical care professional or a dietician.

Illnesses Caused by Food Allergy

As you try to determine if your pain and discomfort may be caused by food allergy, ask yourself a question: Could my symptoms be caused by food allergy? To answer this question you need to know the symptoms that food allergy causes. I will try to answer this question.

It's not easy. Describing the illnesses caused by food allergy is like trying to gift-wrap an elephant—there's not enough paper to do it. What's more, even if you had enough paper, where would you start?

I know this analogy is a little ridiculous, but it does give you some idea of the dilemma I faced in writing this section. Food allergy provokes so many illnesses that to include an elaborate scientific description of all of them would have made this book so expensive the average person couldn't afford to buy it—or carry it.

Besides that, I did not write this book to help you diagnose your own illnesses. Diagnosing and treating illnesses should be left to your medical care professional, and you should not rely on any book to diagnose yourself. Your medical caregiver is trained to recognize symptoms and determine their cause. Go to her or him for help so you can avoid the mistakes that will surely result from self-diagnosis and treatment.

Instead, the purpose of this book is simply to make you more conscious of food allergy and the many illnesses associated with it, as well as to let you know that your symptoms may be caused by food allergy. In this section I want to increase your awareness of these symptoms. If you suffer from any of these symptoms, you should at least consider the possibility that they are food-related.

Direct and indirect causes. The long list of disorders for which food allergy is the direct cause is augmented by numerous illnesses for which it is indirectly responsible. Like an inconsiderate bully, allergy delights in the opportunity to further torment my patients who suffer nonallergic disease.

For instance, we often see patients with back pain caused by degenerated vertebrae or whiplash injury; food allergy greatly intensifies this pain. For patients with intestinal inflammations such as ulcerative colitis, allergy makes their bouts of painful diarrhea more offensive. In these instances, the disorder is not directly caused by food allergy; food is aggravating a preexisting condition.

In the following summary of allergic illnesses, I will not make a point of telling you which illnesses allergy affects directly and which indirectly. Since doctors are unsure of the cause of many illnesses, it is not always possible to make that distinction. However, it is important to realize that if exposure to certain foods causes discomfort and pain, you must avoid them.

Allergic Illnesses: Blood Vessels

The blood vessels are an appropriate place to begin our exploration of the illnesses brought on by food allergy. So many allergic symptoms can be explained in part or altogether by swelling or spasm of the blood vessels and how this swelling stimulates the sensations of itch, or by swelling arising from the nerves that interact with these blood vessels. Food allergy can cause these vessels to swell or spasm.

Migraine Headaches
A popular theory holds that migraine headaches arise from spasms of the blood vessels in the head. The spasm restricts blood flow, denying blood-borne nutrition and oxygen to the brain and eyes. This decrease in energy and oxygen produces the vision changes and numbness that warn many patients they are about to be socked with migraine's agonizing pain.

These headaches may be caused by a vulnerability of the nervous system to sudden changes in either your body or the environment around you. Many researchers believe that migraine sufferers have inherited a more sensitive nervous-system response than those without migraines. During a migraine attack, changes in the activity of the nerves controlling the blood vessels that surround the outside of the brain inflame these blood vessels.

The controller nerves force the blood vessels into spasm. The migraine head pain erupts when the blood vessels relax after the spasm is over. Unfortunately, they relax too much and swell like a boiling sausage, stretching and irritating the nerves that connect the blood vessels to the pain-sensing areas of the brain. Then, when blood circulates through these vessels, pushed by the pumping of the beating heart, each pulse of blood further irritates these pain-sensing nerve fibers, giving the characteristic pain of a migraine headache that pulses in time with the heartbeat.

Hives and Angioedema

Another disorder that we can explain by blood vessel changes is hives, a condition characterized by intensely itchy red blotches—some large, some small—caused by the swelling of small blood vessels at the surface of the skin. The swollen vessels leak fluid into the surrounding skin, causing the skin to swell into a welt and turn red.

The discomfort that accompanies the hives results from irritation of the itch-sensitive nerves at the skin's surface. Not only are hives uncomfortable, they also can be terribly embarrassing. Imagine going to work with red splotches all over your face! Many patients have suffered that experience.

Angioedema is a condition in which the hives form deep in the skin. Patients develop swelling that can turn fingers into sausages, raise flat-topped welts on the skin, and puff up the eyelids, hands, and feet. These deep-seated swellings, which are sometimes redder and sometimes paler than the surrounding skin, typically do not itch because the nerve fibers at the surface of the skin are not stimulated to send out an itch sensation. Often hives and angioedema strike together, and patients suffer both the red, itchy hives and the uncomfortable swelling.

Asthma

Blood vessel changes also can explain some characteristics of asthma, which causes difficulty in clearing air from the lungs. During severe asthma attacks, the chests of victims become distended because their breath is trapped in their lungs like the air in an overinflated balloon. In severe attacks of asthma, exhaling, which is second nature to all of us, becomes an exhausting struggle.

Breathing is difficult because the passages that carry air to the far reaches of the lungs are obstructed. The blood vessels swell and leak fluid into the airway lining, much as they do in hives and angioedema. The swollen linings partially block the passage of air, producing the irritating and sometimes frightening whistle or wheezing sound so familiar in asthma sufferers.

The same swelling that causes migraine headaches, hives and angioedema, and asthma occurs in a number of other areas. We'll examine the consequences of this reaction in the respiratory tract, the sinuses, the chest, and the joints.

Swelling in the Respiratory Tract

If the swelling centers in the vocal cords, it makes the voice *hoarse;* further swelling results in *voice loss.* This happens frequently in many patients; it especially handicaps singers, ministers, and others who frequently address the public. Perhaps the strain these activities put on the vocal cords weakens the area and makes the vocal cords more susceptible to allergy's voice changes.

Swelling in an area near the vocal cords, especially when accompanied by an annoying itch in the breathing passages, brings on the *chronic cough* and persistent *throat irritation* that exasperate so many patients. The spring and fall rainy seasons send a constant stream of coughing and throat-clearing patients to allergists, usually at the request of parents, spouses, or friends who tire of listening to this irritating, barking cough day and night.

For a sizable share of the population, the airway swelling becomes so pronounced that they feel like they are strangling. The strangling feeling, I believe, arises from a *swelling of the airway*—a swelling that makes patients feel they cannot breathe. Fortunately in most people the strangling feeling does not progress to real strangulation because the airway swelling causes only a partial blockage. Although this is almost always a harmless symptom, patients often live in fear that one of these attacks will be their last.

Medical care professionals often may misdiagnose this frightening disorder and call it *hyperventilation*, a diagnosis implying an anxiety origin. This is not necessarily so.

There are clues that this choking feeling is real and not imagined. Patients who suffer from airway swelling usually know that it is real—that something is blocking their breathing. They even point to the spot on the neck or the chest where they feel the obstruction.

Although their struggle for air is similar to the hyperventilation that accompanies anxiety attacks, and they are anxious during the attack, their anxiety is brought on by the feeling of strangulation and not the psyche. Forget the tranquilizers!

When the swelling occurs higher in the respiratory tract, its symptoms are relatively harmless but unpleasant. If the swelling is at the back of the throat, it can cause a *recurrent sore throat*. Although painful, these sore throats seem to have no infectious basis because they produce negative throat cultures. The throat usually looks normal on examination.

It can also produce *swelling of the tongue, lips, or membranes in the mouth*, as well as the most common complaint of allergy patients—*nasal stuffiness*. This unpleasant symptom, which results from swelling in the mucous membranes of the nose, is like having a constant cold with its accompanying tiredness, irritability, and just plain yuckiness. It is frustrating to treat this condition if the patient refuses to limit the foods and beverages that promote the stuffiness.

Swelling in the Sinuses

If the swelling is even higher in the respiratory tract—in the sinuses—patients experience the nagging, steady pressure and pain of *sinus headaches*. More than half of the patients who come to allergists for treatment feel aggravating pain in the forehead, eyes, cheeks, or back of the head that is characteristic of these distressing headaches. I know firsthand how distressful they can be; I suffered dreadful sinus headaches. The opportunity to help others avoid these headaches attracted me to the field of allergy.

Swelling in the Chest

Another surprisingly common allergic symptom is *chest pain*. My patients often complain of a painful tightening or a heavy sensation under the sternum (breastbone), much like that experienced by people suffering a heart attack. There can even be changes in the rhythm of the heart, either speeding it up or slowing it down, and at times caus-ing missed beats. More than a few doctors have been surprised to see a normal EKG in a patient suffering allergic chest pain.

Swelling in the Joints

Allergy torments weak or damaged areas; it is no surprise that the swelling of angioedema frequently attacks the muscles and joints of patients with nonallergy-related diseases such as rheumatoid arthritis or osteoarthritis. The swelling generally occurs deep in the affected joints; you do not see it on the surface of the joint, nor do you feel the heat or redness that are the hallmarks of arthritic inflammation. Many of my patients with arthritis experience episodes of pain in their arthritic joints when they cheat on my diet.

This same annoying pain bothers joints that have been damaged by injury. Patients with whiplash and other spine injury are vulnerable, as well as those with temporomandibular joint (TMJ) syndrome or post-traumatic joint injury (e.g., joints damaged by football injury). Here again I speak from personal experience. My "football" knee aches and swells with fluid when I exceed my tolerance for certain foods—in my case, almost always those flavored by MSG (monosodium glutamate), blundered into by mistake.

Nerves, Blood Vessels, and Mystery

Much of the mystery surrounding allergies stems from their ability to strike widely separated areas of the body, areas as unrelated as the joints and the respiratory tract. But in the previous discussion I used a key bit of information to dispel this mystery.

We saw how widely separated and unrelated parts of the body are affected by the same process—irritation and spasm of blood vessels. In tracking this swelling as it moved around the body, we learned why allergic disorders bring widespread discomfort and pain. We also saw that allergy targets areas already weakened by injury or disease as well as areas genetically predisposed to allergy's miseries.

Understanding swelling and multiple affected areas, we know that allergy is not mysterious. To further dispel its apparent mysteries, let's further explore the relationship between blood vessels and nerves and see how this relationship leads to symptoms caused by the overload of dietary chemicals.

Blood vessels can no more dilate or spasm by themselves than a car can drive itself. Imagine picking up the morning paper and reading: MR. JONES'S 1990 HUPMOBILE JAILED AFTER BEING CONVICTED OF SMASHING INTO STOP SIGN.

Upon reading this, you would feel that you should probably make reservations for the reporter, the judge, and the arresting officer at the nearest psychiatric ward and order a trial for Mr. Jones, the car's driver. The car is not at fault, the driver is.

Just as cars do not drive themselves, so blood vessels do not order themselves to dilate. Nerves do the ordering; they manipulate the blood vessels, making them swell and spasm. Understanding this nerve/blood vessel relationship is key to understanding how allergy plagues the nerves and blood vessels.

There is evidence that certain foods damage nerves and that these damaged nerves stimulate blood vessels to swell and leak. Nerves are stimulated by neurotransmitters (i.e., chemicals that transmit or carry messages to nerves). Some of the foods we will discuss are neurostimulating and neurotoxic (i.e., damaging to nerves). It is possible that these foods directly stimulate the nerves that govern blood vessels, forcing dilatation and swelling and provoking food-sensitive patients' discomfort and pain.

Allergic Illnesses: Smooth Muscles

Blood vessels are not the only body tissues involved in allergic illnesses. Muscles called "smooth muscles" also participate. The smooth muscles we are concerned with encircle the digestive tract and the airways of the lung.

I visualize allergy's effect on smooth muscles as the same effect it exerts on blood vessels. Like the vessels, smooth muscles are richly supplied with nerves, and these nerves "drive" smooth muscles like we drive a car. Also like blood vessels, nerve impulses force smooth muscles to spasm or relax. Unlike the vessels, which cause allergic illness by relaxation (swelling), smooth muscles cause pain when they spasm or contract.

Asthma
In looking at asthma earlier, we saw that blood vessel swelling in the lining of the airways constricts the air passages, obstructing the flow of

air and causing the whistling or wheezing sound we hear as the air forces itself out of these narrowed air passages. But we shouldn't limit our discussion to swelling of the lining because that is not the only reason the air passages constrict.

Each air passage is surrounded by layers of muscle, the smooth muscle we are examining, just as the water running to a sprinkler is surrounded by the walls of a hose. Unlike the rigid walls of a hose, the muscle around the air passages is alive and in constant motion. It dilates and contracts to open or to close the numerous branches of the airway, directing the flow of air to different parts of the lung like a traffic officer directs the flow of traffic through a busy intersection.

What if during rush hour, the traffic officer went on strike, closing half of each road leading into the intersection? Pandemonium would result, with angry, snarling drivers trapped in a gridlock. The stream of traffic would be slowed almost to a halt, and it would take forever for the cars to thread their way through the intersection.

Asthma is like that. Things go smoothly when the airway muscle is functioning normally, contracting and relaxing as it calmly directs the flow of air. When the muscle is in spasm during an asthma attack, the airway narrows, restricting the flow of air through the intersections of the lung.

Food allergy is only one of many causes of asthma attacks, but when diet is involved, the most likely reason is nerve malfunction causing swelling and signaling the smooth muscle of the airways to go into spasm. The swelling further causes the muscles to spasm. Dietary discretion can reduce this spasm the same way it controls the blood vessel swelling in the lining of the airway.

Smooth-Muscle Spasm Along the Digestive Tract

When spasm occurs in the stomach, it is referred to as acid stomach or *esophageal reflux* and often leads patients to suspect that they have an ulcer. Those who do have ulcers are especially susceptible to this condition, another example of allergy preying on an already weakened area. The combination of food allergy and ulcer produces a persistent, gnawing pain. Unfortunately, changing the diet will not cure an ulcer, but it can eliminate this aggravating complication.

At the end of the intestine, and surrounded by the same smooth muscle, is the colon, an organ frequently affected by allergy. Here muscle spasms give rise to the *abdominal cramps and diarrhea* that so often make my patients' lives miserable. Doctors often diagnose these symptoms as spastic colon or irritable bowel. In many cases, food allergy is not suspected; however, changing the diet usually alleviates these cramps and diarrhea.

Allergic Illnesses: Contact Dermatitis

Our trip through the digestive tract ends at the rectum, where an uncommon but miserable effect of food chemicals manifests itself. A small number of allergy-prone adults complain of an intense *rectal itching* that mystifies doctors.

The acid foods seem unusually adept at causing this uncomfortable and embarrassing condition, although other foods also contribute. *Diaper rash* in babies is more common and often is caused by these same offenders. I suspect that as the stool passes through the anus, a high concentration of acid from foods irritates and burns the skin.

We know that this contact reaction occurs at the other end of the body, where patients suffer *scalp rash* marked by itching and sores from using shampoos that contain citrus.

Another form of contact dermatitis that should be mentioned is the oh-so-common *hand dermatitis*, sometimes called housewife's hand dermatitis. Anyone who handles acidic foods is susceptible. Contact with these foods makes hands red, dry, cracked, and very itchy.

Allergic Illnesses: Central Nervous System

The effect of food allergy on the central nervous system—the brain—is perhaps the most difficult subject to discuss because it is surrounded by uncertainty and controversy. Many doctors and laypeople do not accept the idea that food chemicals can impair brain function or be responsible for the many symptoms that patients suffer. They believe that anxiety, depression, and other mood disorders are more likely to be at the root of these symptoms.

I disagree. As we examine our modern diet, I will point out that certain components are known neurotoxins (e.g., aspartic and glutamic acids), and I will give you a theory about how they and other food chemicals can generate allergic disease through injury to nerves. Do we

suddenly reverse our thinking when it comes to the major nerve center
of the body, the brain, and say it cannot be affected? I see no reason to
do so.

At the same time, I don't want you to think that foods are solely or
even primarily responsible for these disorders. Anxiety and psychological instability are often major causes. In other cases they may be contributing factors that potentiate allergy's harm. To illustrate this point,
think of food allergy in some people as driving these illnesses like a
hammer drives a nail. In other people it seems to play more of a sup-
portive role, like the fingers holding the nail. But whatever the relative
contribution of each factor, an allergist's job is to help his or her patients
gain relief, and changing the diet often provides some of that relief.

Perhaps the best way I can illustrate the effects of food allergy on mental function is through one of my patient histories. Frequently I see
patients who complain of allergic symptoms that are so minor I wonder
why my patients came for treatment. When I ask them how they feel in
general, the real reason comes tumbling out. They tell me about being
tired, irritable, and depressed all the time—just plain feeling crummy
and unable to cope with everyday life. Jackie is one of those patients.

Jackie is a woman in her forties who serves as a middle manager in a
nationally known company. She had been feeling tired and listless for
so long she was worried about her ineffectiveness at work. "I had my
doctor check my thyroid because I was sure I was hypothyroid, but the
tests were normal. Then I began to think that I was 'wimping out'—
that the tiredness was all in my head."

"That's not at all unusual, Jackie," I assured her. "It isn't necessarily
all in your head. Many people find that physical factors, such as food
allergy, cause these symptoms."

Jackie's symptoms are almost as frequent in my patients as stuffy
nose or headache. What's more, patients often hide these symptoms as
they would hide a disgraceful family secret. Like Jackie, they are afraid
to "wimp out" because they don't want to be thought of as a hypochon-
driac—a whiner and a complainer. They are not any of these things.
Tiredness, irritability, and often hyperactivity and the inability to concentrate frequently accompany food allergy and usually subside with
diet changes.

When Jackie returned to my office after her first three months of treatment, I remember our conversation. I asked, "How are you doing, Jackie?"

"Changing my diet helped much more than I thought it would, Dr. Walsh," she reported. "I know you asked me to retry the foods I've eliminated, but I feel so good, I'm afraid to return to them.

"I'm surprised at how much better I feel. I'm not as tired, and I've got a lot more ambition at work. Although I'm not 100 percent better, I have improved so much I no longer think it's all in my head."

Then Jackie told me that she made another interesting discovery. "I was talking to one of my coworkers the other day. She told me she sees you, too, and has to follow the same diet. Every time she cheats, she ends up feeling tired and irritable and her work suffers."

Since then, Jackie finds that her ability to concentrate at work nose-dives when she strays from the diet she should follow, a symptom shared by many of my patients. They have difficulty describing this familiar effect of foods, but many agree that an appropriate label would be "spacey" thinking.

You might think I go too far—that foods we have eaten all our lives can't possibly affect our mental ability—but don't be too sure. We are learning that the thought and memory processes that take place in the brain are assisted and influenced by neurotransmitters. Some of the foods we will discuss contain appreciable levels of these neurotransmitters, and you do not need to stretch your imagination far to reason that, in certain susceptible people, they may muddle thinking and turn it "spacey."

Neurotransmitters are a hot research topic in the study of depression. Since allergy and depression both appear frequently in our modern society, it isn't surprising that they often coexist in patients.

Food allergy does not cause depression, but the tiredness, irritability, and ineffective thinking that often accompany food allergy can make depression much harder to overcome. Modifying the diet helps to relieve these symptoms. Depressed patients who also suffer from allergy deserve the same allergy care as those who are free of depression.

Other Allergic Illnesses
Although I have described many discomforts and pains of patients, there are still many others I have not included that may affect you.

Describing every possible symptom would make this section too long. Every day patients tell allergists of aches, pains, and discomforts brought on by allergy, many strange and unusual, all a burden. If you suffer from these symptoms, I hope I can help you avoid the foods that cause them.

We have examined the illnesses caused by food allergy. If it causes so many illnesses, you must wonder why it is so difficult to diagnose. Let's explore this topic next as we look at an overview of food allergy and the complications encountered in its diagnosis.

Overview of Food Allergy and Complications in Diagnosing Food Allergy

The ways in which people react to foods vary as much as the ways by which they eat this food. They can gulp the food quickly or eat it leisurely, hastily satisfy their hunger, or enjoy a lazy meal.

As people eat, so can they react to foods. They can react quickly and dramatically and then recover equally rapidly—or become sick slowly and recover sluggishly. This difference in the quickness of reactions to food confuses many food-sensitive people and often hides the food allergy that causes their illness.

Other factors compound this confusion. As the speed of the reaction can vary, so can the number of foods involved—one food or many foods may bring pain and discomfort. The involved foods can be obvious and the patient sure of the cause, or the identity of these foods obscure and the sufferer confused.

For some, symptoms strike when they consume even a minuscule amount of food; others need a comparatively large quantity before experiencing pain and discomfort. On skin testing, the harmful foods may surface, or perversely hide their identity.

With all these confusing factors, you can see why diagnosis can be complicated for these poor food sufferers. Let's try to help you understand these factors by examining the variances I just mentioned, one at a time.

Sudden, Dramatic Food Reactions

For many people, even tiny amounts of such foods as nuts, fish, peanuts, and shellfish can precipitate severe and life-threatening illnesses; because they are quick-striking and dramatic, a person's attention is immediately drawn to the food. The sufferer usually does not have trouble determining the culprit food.

An example of this type of allergy is the person who dines at a nice restaurant, enjoying a delectable meal of shrimp. Suddenly his eyes swell and tears flow, his nasal passages close, his skin erupts with angry red hives, and his air passage swells, threatening to strangle him. The reaction is dramatic, frightening, and dangerous. Obvious cause—shrimp. Obvious response—no more shrimp!

Allergy to a Single Food

As the example of the shrimp reaction shows, the quickness and severity of dangerous food reactions startle the victim and forcibly grab his or her attention. The culprit food is even easier to identify when only one food is responsible. Then the quick-appearing reaction points directly to this food. If you experience diarrhea or hives every time you eat corn or carrots, you know where the problem lies.

Infrequently consumed foods are easier to spot than those eaten more frequently. However, in many cases a commonly consumed food such as wheat, or a beverage such as milk, is at fault. Because the food is eaten at every meal, it's hard to pinpoint because the symptoms continue without letup or return daily. Then, a nonallergic illness such as an inflammation to the intestines or arthritis is suspected and the true cause—food—is ignored.

Allergy to Multiple Foods

As the number of foods causing symptoms multiplies, the difficulty in finding these foods also multiplies. When a person eats or drinks a number of potentially harmful foods at a meal and then suffers symptoms, he or she easily becomes confused.

Although the patient with one food allergy seldom needs help finding the food, the patient with many food allergies often needs help.

Genny, a fifty-five-year-old mother of four and grandmother of three, had been sent to me by her internist after years of struggling unsuccessfully to treat her daily abdominal pains and crippling migraine headaches. Her symptoms began after her second child was born and often made the demanding role of motherhood a dreadful ordeal. In fact, pain often forced her to take to her bed, even when her children were small and needed supervision. She was miserable.

As I investigated her food allergies I found she suffered from multiple and serious food allergies. When I considered how to treat her, I admit I was discouraged. However, we pursued our usual approach to the patient with multiple food allergies, the approach we will be discussing as we proceed in our exploration of food allergy.

It worked! Genny returned to see me in three months, with both abdominal pain and migraines markedly improved. No days spent in bed. My staff and I were delighted.

There are many people like Genny in our practice, each with his or her own pitiful tale. With each patient I worry whether I can control these truly troublesome multiple-food allergies; with almost all patients I find that the tools of the allergist—combined with the patient's fine cooperation and hard work—bring about a pleasing reduction of miserable symptoms.

Slow-Developing Food Reactions

Now the diagnosis of food allergy becomes even more difficult. We no longer have the guidance of the fast-striking food reaction (i.e., eat shrimp, get immediately sick). To further confuse diagnosis, most of the patients in my practice with slow-developing food allergies react to multiple foods; they suffer all the puzzlement that multiple food allergy brings.

For instance, Linda is a forty-two-year-old printing salesperson who must often entertain her clients at restaurants. She never develops symptoms after dinner, but the next morning she wakes up feeling crummy. Her hands and stomach bloat, and her bathroom scale records extra pounds of fluid; her cramps and diarrhea force her to stay home from the office, or she tries to go to work but suffers a miserable day; she is tired, irritable, and understandably depressed.

Linda came to see me because she couldn't understand why eating out caused such severe symptoms. She is a bright woman, so lack of mental ability didn't prevent her from recognizing the cause of her symptoms. Because it took hours for her suffering to begin, the harmful foods were concealed, they were multiple, and their effects appeared slowly.

Fortunately, we were able to single out the offending foods, and as long as Linda avoids them, she awakens refreshed in the morning.

By now you have some understanding of the roadblocks allergists encounter in diagnosing slow-developing and multiple-food allergies. You might think these are the only factors that slow allergists as we try to solve the mysteries of our patients' miseries. I wish you were right. Another important factor hinders our diagnosis: accumulation, and its role in concealing the foods that cause illness.

Accumulation

Most of us can identify with accumulation in the usual sense of the word. Remember that Thanksgiving dinner when you stuffed yourself until you felt like your stomach would burst? You just plain ate too much! You loosened your belt while berating yourself for eating like a pig. You accumulated too much food, and the accumulated food brought you discomfort because of the sheer bulk in your stomach.

If you have food allergy, accumulation doesn't mean eating an amount of food so massive that your stomach bloats and your belt pinches. It means eating or drinking too much of the foods or beverages you tolerate poorly. Foods or beverages that won't hurt you in small quantities will bring pain and discomfort if you exceed that magic amount your body can handle.

Accumulation does not occur in most of the quick-striking and dangerous food allergies. In these reactions, often only a small amount of food is necessary to bring illness, sometimes only the minuscule amount you breathe when you smell it cooking. This same small amount triggers many single-food allergies and some of the multiple-food allergies. In these cases, accumulation is not a factor; my patients can't tolerate any of the offending food or foods.

However, with most cases of slow-reacting and multiple-food allergies, accumulative-food allergy is important. Because many people suffer slow-reacting and multiple-food allergy, accumulation commonly accompanies food allergy. Many of my patients can tolerate some offending food, but any quantity above this tolerance level leads to misfortune.

Although many quick-striking food reactions are dangerous and even deadly, those associated with accumulation usually aren't. Although they frequently bring pain and discomfort, they seldom threaten life. Although this relative lack of danger is an advantage, the difficulty in diagnosing these reactions isn't. Unlike quick-striking food reactions, accumulative reactions require a lot of detective work that can be frustrating and perplexing.

The Additive Effect

The additive effect of food allergy further complicates its diagnosis. This additive effect accompanies multiple-food allergies. Eating a small amount of a number of offending foods (additive effect) is the same as eating a large amount of one food. For instance, if too much orange juice makes your stomach cramp, you might think you can solve the problem by drinking only one little glassful a day.

It's not that easy. If you don't realize that strawberries and tomatoes, for example, reinforce the painful effects of orange juice, and you consume some of those foods in addition to a little orange juice, your stomach will continue cramping and you will continue aching, discouraged because you feel you missed the diagnosis.

Don't give up; there may be a number of foods, acting in combination, causing your stomach ache. If you find one of them (e.g., orange juice), don't stop thinking and investigating. Look for brother and sister foods that add to the distressing cramping caused by orange juice. Eating less of all these foods should calm your stomach.

Accumulation and Addition and the Onset of Symptoms

How soon after a meal will symptoms strike? How long does it take to fill a bucket? The answers are the same. If the bucket is empty, it may take a long time to fill it. If it is full, it may slop over if you add a single drop of water. Managing accumulative food allergy is the same as adding no more to the bucket than the amount withdrawn daily.

If you suffer from food allergy and eat an offending food, it may take hours or up to a day or more for illness to strike—or you may not even get sick—if you haven't eaten other offending foods lately. In this case, you don't have enough of these foods accumulated in your body to cause symptoms. You would not be adding more to your bucket than what it holds.

However, if you ate enough of these foods lately, you would be like that full bucket that can't hold even a tiny bit more water—you could react quickly. That's why many people find that the time from eating to onset of symptoms varies. It can range from minutes to hours to days, a variation that can confuse you.

Time of onset also varies depending on the amount consumed. A little bit may be okay—no symptoms. A larger amount may cause a mild reaction the next day. A meal featuring lots of an aggravating food forces early and severe discomfort. Even more variability and more confusion.

I am reminded of Mike's case of migraine headaches. Mike owned a local franchise of a major restaurant chain, so his attention was naturally directed to foods as a possible cause for his migraines. But Mike was confused. Sometimes he was sure certain foods caused the migraines; the pain struck right after he ate them. Sometimes he was sure they didn't; he ate them without experiencing pain or the headache appeared the next day. When his neurologist couldn't explain these odd circumstances, he sent Mike to see me.

The answer lay in his story. Mike was affected by multiple foods, his symptoms appeared only after he had accumulated enough to have a headache, the foods were additive in their effects, and all of this brought variability to the time of onset of his headache pain.

When we identified the group of foods that caused his migraines and explained why he experienced variability in his symptoms, Mike was able to avoid food-caused migraine headaches. As long as he doesn't cheat on his diet (as he does at times), food doesn't give him headaches.

Craving: A Factor without Explanation

Another factor that interferes with the diagnosis of food allergy is craving. It seems ironic that many humans crave the foods that harm them. Food craving often blocks a patient from accepting an allergist's advice on which foods to avoid.

I suspect that the craving factor is operating when a patient tells his or her allergist, "I can't believe these foods cause me any problems." Or, "That can't be right. These foods don't bother me." These are characteristic responses from patients with food cravings who don't want to even consider the possibility that the foods they love cause their discomfort.

You might wonder why I believe that this is a form of denial in certain patients. The answer is simple. After they admit that these foods really harm them—typically about three years later—they also admit that their food cravings made them reject our advice. (I don't know why it so often takes three years, but it does.)

Past and Present Training and Conditioning

Another factor interfering with the diagnosis of food allergy is past and present training and conditioning. We are conditioned to believe that certain foods are healthy; we are persuaded that we must eat them every day because they are essential; we are convinced that without them our diets are unhealthy. Mama told us, teacher told us, and now dieticians and other health experts tell us that we must eat these foods. Unfortunately, for those who suffer allergy, Mama, teacher, and dieticians were and are mistaken.

Even though we know they are mistaken, it is hard for us to discard this well-intentioned advice. Each of the foods and food chemicals we will discuss in this book are defended vociferously by acknowledged experts in food science who honestly believe they are safe. Some of these foods are regarded as essential to a healthy diet. Many scientific studies confirm the conclusions of these experts. Unfortunately, some patients' reactions to these foods deny their value and safety.

This lifelong conditioning is the reason why so many folks with allergies continue to consume the foods and beverages that cause distress: "After all," they tell themselves, "orange juice has a lot of vitamin C." This conditioning is also the reason why so many medical professionals are unaware of the illness or illnesses that certain foods can cause some patients with allergies: "Can't be milk. It's such an important source of calcium." And it's also the reason a patient often resists an allergist's advice: "Can't be wheat. Mother always said bread was the staff of life."

Prior and present conditioning definitely complicate the diagnosis and treatment of food allergy. So many people find it ridiculous even to suspect that the glassful of orange juice clutched in their fist packs not only vitamins but also a lot of misery. Persuading them otherwise is often quite a job.

It's Not Hopeless

With this lengthy discussion of the complexity of food allergy, you may think I am telling you that diagnosis is hopeless. I am not. You can learn to diagnose your own food allergy.

Speaking as an allergist, I admit that I could easily fail to diagnose or help food-sensitive patients, but in most cases I succeed because food allergy has one helpful trait. Each food (or group of foods) tends to cause characteristic symptoms; not all the time, but enough times to help identify the food. After years of diagnosing and treating food allergy, a doctor can use this tendency to help his or her patients. I hope this book will help you learn these characteristic reactions so you can use that knowledge.

Another factor making the diagnosis and treatment of food allergy possible is that certain foods, beverages, and food chemicals are the worst offenders. If you know them, this knowledge will guide you to discovering their role in your illness. When you look for them, you will find the food allergies we already discussed: they may involve multiple foods, be accumulative or additive, their symptoms may be variable in time of onset, or patients may often crave them.

Once a person with symptoms recognizes and determines his or her tolerance for these foods, a lot of the mystery surrounding food allergy disappears.

How Allergy Starts

In the next few sections we will discuss thoughts and principles that will guide you as you look for signs of food allergy in your own symptoms. They are the same thoughts and principles that I teach medical care professionals who visit my office.

For many years these doctors and other medical care providers have joined me in my office to learn how to treat allergic patients. I welcome them and enjoy their visits. Seeing the dawn of understanding light up their faces as they start to understand the terrible burden imposed on patients by allergy is a great reward. I know that the knowledge I give them will help these professionals more effectively treat their own patients, will guide them to the path improving their patient's health. Their understanding of allergy is one of the most rewarding aspects of my practice.

We will begin our exploration of food allergy in the same way I begin teaching the medical care professionals who visit me in my office. Before seeing patients, we find a quiet room and review some general principles I use to diagnose and treat food allergy.

We will start with my first and most important principle: *You cannot treat your allergy if you do not suspect it*

You're probably thinking, "Gee, that seems obvious—and wouldn't it be true of any illness?"

But allergy isn't like any other illness. In many cases it lacks its own clear-cut set of symptoms and, instead, mimics those of other illnesses. That's why it is important for you to take this principle to heart. If you fail to suspect allergy as a possible cause of the symptoms you suffer, you will not seek allergy care, nor will you find and eliminate the foods and environmental conditions that make you ill. Suspecting allergy is your first step on the road to good health.

This first step is not an obvious one for many people. For you it may be obvious—your suspicion of allergy caused you to read this book. But think back to how your allergy symptoms started. They might have crept quietly into your life like a silent predator, to steal your comfort and replace it with pain and discomfort. Like a pickpocket stealing your wallet, it tried to avoid getting caught. Often it hides under a cloak of confusion, making it difficult for you to suspect it. Perhaps the best example of this confusion is the sneaky way it often starts.

Allergy Often Starts like a Cold

Allergy often starts like a simple, virus-caused cold. Prior to its onset you feel fine—no sneezing, wheezing, or itching. But one day you begin to notice those old, familiar symptoms of a cold. Your spirits droop, you cough, your chest feels tight, and your head aches. Then your nose begins to drip, your head totally stuffs up, and that tickle in your throat turns into a raspy cough. Once again you have fallen victim to the common cold virus. Having survived many colds, you know just what to do. Take it easy, drink plenty of liquids, get lots of rest, and wait for the cold to slip quietly out of your life.

However, this time it's different. Instead of clearing up in a few days, your symptoms go on and on. Week after week, month after month, the symptoms wax and wane. At times you feel a little better; at other times your nose is so stuffy and your head so painful that routine tasks become a chore. Your doctor treats you for a sinus infection, but the sinus pains return soon after you finish the antibiotic. Your "cold" won't leave, and you don't know why.

Patty and Michelle serve as good examples of allergy following on the heels of a cold. Patty's mom, a local physician, called me about her daughter. She was suffering with huge red hives that started on her arms and spread to cover her entire body; they itched so much that at night she tossed and turned, sleeping only fitfully.

She told me that Patty was not eating shrimp, peanuts, or other hive-causing foods when the hives began. Although she was not eating them when the hives started, she must now avoid them—they seem to make her hives worse. This is surprising—Patty had never reacted to them in the past. The most likely explanation is that a virus infection like the common cold caused the hives; they first appeared while she was recovering from a cold that had made the rounds of the family. As the virus departed, it left the hives behind. Now that the hives are present, she must identify and avoid the foods that make the hives flare up.

Michelle's story is similar. Ever since she suffered a severe viral cold, with pneumonia, Michelle has wheezed. Wheezing showing up after a virus-caused cold is common among my patients with asthma and shows the ability of a virus to initiate asthma. Now that the asthma is present, Michelle must avoid foods and environmental exposures that make her wheeze. Combining Michelle's story with the large number of patients whose hives started after a cold leaves little doubt that viruses often are the keys that unlock allergic illness.

Too Much Musty Air Can Trigger Allergy

Allergy symptoms may also start for reasons that are unrelated to virus infections. For example, although most of us know that pollen triggers allergy, few realize that other environmental factors do the same. A home with too many house dust mites and too much mold, yeast, and algae can start allergy symptoms.

For instance, Becky and Jim came into my office for evaluation. Becky was suffering from frequent and painful headaches, and Jim complained of nasal stuffiness. Their symptoms started soon after they moved into their current home. Even though this home is on a hill, which should ensure that rainwater drains safely away from the foundation, the basement still leaks water with each rain. It smells musty and must be moldy—a good reason why both Becky and Jim are miserable.

Another example of the environment's role in initiating allergy is Jeanine's daughter, Kris. Every day at school she suffers migraine headaches and often spends more that an hour in the nurse's office. A number of teachers from that school also are my patients—suffering the same headaches as their students. Unfortunately, they can't afford to spend an hour in the nurse's office every day.

Many other examples come readily to mind, including that of Mary, whose cough started after steam-cleaning her carpets (introducing mold with the water?) or that of Pat, whose stuffy nose started after remodeling his daughter's old house (was the wood he was sawing moldy?). If Becky, Jim, Jeanine, Mary, or Pat had not recognized school, work, or home as the source of illness, they would not have suspected allergy.

Allergy Can Start for No Known Reason

Perhaps one day you feel stomach cramps and notice that your stools are loose. At first you suspect that you've caught a stomach flu, but instead of disappearing in a day or two, your cramps and diarrhea return again and again. When your symptoms start, you wonder if you have fallen prey to some foodborne bacteria. When your symptoms continue, you start suspecting allergy.

On the other hand, allergy may begin with a bout of sneezing and an itchy nose. Your nose has never bothered you quite this way before, but it feels uncomfortable now. You chalk up your discomfort to a mild cold or sinus infection and decide not to worry. It should go away by tomorrow. But it doesn't go away tomorrow, the next day, or the next week; you start suspecting allergy.

No matter how your allergic symptoms start, they confuse you because they do not seem to have a specific cause. Why won't your cold go away? Why does your stomach ache, your head hurt, or your skin itch? You've never suffered from allergy to anything in your life, so why should you suspect allergy now, especially at your age?

Unfortunately, although you are confused by allergy starting in such a bewildering way, and at an age you do not expect, your allergy may be causing your symptoms. You cannot seek proper care until you realize that fact.

To further confuse the issue, allergy attacks many different parts of your body. Is it possible that allergy can make your stomach hurt, your skin itch, your joints ache, and your sleep fitful, all at the same time? Aren't these totally different symptoms caused by totally different illnesses? You haven't changed anything in your house or eaten any new foods, so how can allergy bother you?

If I am to succeed at teaching you to treat your own food allergies, you should know that multiple symptoms are possible. Only then can you strip away the confusion that hides allergy—the true cause of your symptoms.

Two mistaken beliefs are major roadblocks to suspecting allergy. I will discuss them next, so they do not interfere with your ability to suspect that allergy causes your pain and discomfort.

Age and Diet: Factors in Food Allergy

My patients often ask me two questions:

1. "I didn't have allergy before. Why should it bother me now?"
2. "I haven't changed my diet. How could I be allergic to certain foods?"

These questions tell me that my patients had a mistaken view of allergy that prevented them from discovering that it caused their symptoms, needlessly prolonging the time when they finally suspected it and acted on its presence. To prevent you from holding these same mistaken views, I will answer these questions. I will use information that allergists believe to be true and other information that is somewhat speculative but probably true. I will present the proven and speculative information together to help you see allergy as I see it, to assist you in your thinking, and to guide you in your battle against this thief of wellness.

The Age Factor

"I didn't have allergy before. Why should it bother me now?"

It may surprise you that allergy can start at one or at eighty years of age. There is no specific age of onset. Actually, your allergy did not start at one or eighty years of age; your *symptoms* started then. Your allergies were with you when you were born.

Allergy nested in the genes that determine who you are when you emerged from the womb. Your proud mom and pop held a healthy baby but a baby ready, when the right moment arrived, to sneeze, wheeze, or itch. When your symptoms started, at one or eighty or any-where between—that was the right moment.

You did not sneeze, wheeze, or itch in the delivery room because your guardian immune system kept allergy locked inside you. Later in life, when your immune system weakened and could no longer hold your allergy in restraint, your symptoms started.

What weakened your immune system? My experience with patients convinces me that two events we have already discussed weaken your immune system: a virus, or an overwhelming allergy exposure. If we review them now and discuss their effect on the immune system, you will see that age and lack of prior allergic symptoms do not rule out allergy as a cause of your symptoms.

Viruses Weaken Your Immune System

Virus infections can profoundly weaken your immune system. A good example of this weakening occurs in people infected by the AIDS virus. This virus weakens and destroys the lymphocytes of the immune sys-tem, the same lymphocytes that protect against infection. I use the AIDS virus as an example of viruses' potent effect on immunity, not to imply that the viruses that set off allergy have that devastating an effect on the immune system. They do not.

Most viruses do not affect the immune system at all, or weaken it only temporarily. The viruses that start allergy belong to this later, less potent group. They only temporarily weaken the immune system. Unfortunately, "temporarily" can last a long time—weeks to years—before the immune system recovers the strength to overpower allergy, return it to its shackles, and end your symptoms.

Environmental Exposure Also Weakens Your Immune System

Your allergies may start because you lived or worked too long in air contaminated by high levels of dust mite or mold, yeast, and algae. I hear about these exposures frequently in my patients' stories.

Many of my patients lived comfortable lives until they moved into a musty home and stayed too long—or studied for too many years in a musty school or worked too long in a musty building. Under a continuing barrage of house dust mite, mold, yeast, and algae, their immune systems eventually crumbled and allergy escaped. Pain and discomfort followed.

This tie between mustiness and sickness surprises many patients. "But Dr. Walsh, I lived there (or worked or studied there) for three years before my symptoms started."

My reply: "Yes, you did live comfortably for three years, but the air quality was poor, forcing your immune system to carry too heavy a load. Finally, exhausted from fighting too much mustiness too hard for too long, it failed."

Viruses Can Combine with Environmental Exposures

As I listen to my patients tell me about how their allergies began, I hear a recurrent theme—that both environment and virus can join forces to start allergy symptoms.

My patients tell me about living in a musty environment without trouble until they became sick from a cold or other virus infection. Then, headaches, rashes, joint pain, tiredness, and other symptoms of allergy started. In reviewing these stories, I often think that the most potent stimulus to allergy is not virus or exposure but virus *and* exposure.

Allergy Can Start at Birth

If viruses and prolonged harmful environmental exposures cause allergy, does this mean that babies cannot be allergic? After all, their life in the womb shelters them from mite, mold, and pollen, and their mothers' antibodies help them defeat viruses.

I'm afraid the answer to this question is yes, babies can suffer allergies. Sally's story of her son John's stuffiness is typical of many stories. "John was born with a stuffy nose." Allergy truly respects no age, even the tender newborn baby.

Whether weakened by a virus, by prolonged exposure to great mustiness or both, your allergy escaped its immune prison. It now delights in bringing you pain and discomfort. No matter if you are one, twenty, or sixty years of age, the milk, shrimp, or peanuts that you enjoyed without harm yesterday can trouble you today. When you wonder why, remember our first principle and its extension:

Suspect allergy; you cannot treat your allergy if you do not suspect it. Do not think that your age protects you from this bully. It doesn't.

The Diet Factor

"I haven't changed my diet. How could I be allergic to certain foods?"

Now that you have learned to suspect allergy, you wonder if one or more foods may cause your symptoms. They may. To identify them, you might be tempted to concentrate your attention on foods new to your diet. You may be right; new foods cause many allergies. However, if you only pay attention to new foods, you may be making a mistake that seriously interferes with your suspecting allergy. You may find that no new food causes your symptoms and dismiss the thought of allergy.

You could be overlooking the real culprits, foods you have eaten for years. Although we think of these foods as old friends, they may not be friendly at all. As old friends can turn to bitter enemies, so trusted foods can suddenly start to trouble you. Although your diet includes only foods that you have eaten without trouble for years, you may still be food-sensitive—to these same foods in which you invest so much trust.

Why You Now React to Foods You Have Eaten for Years

Yesterday you drank milk and ate wheat, tomatoes, or corn without trouble. However, yesterday is not today, and as the date on the calendar changed, you also changed. You are not the person you were yesterday. When you last ate these foods, you reacted not at all. Today you do react.

In the past your immune system protected you from food allergy—foods could not harm you. Now your immune system no longer protects you from this allergy and you no longer tolerate the foods you ate safely in the past.

Therefore, don't be confused if you fail to identify a new food as the cause of your symptoms. Start suspecting foods that you have eaten without trouble for years.

This leads us to another principle of allergy diagnosis and treatment: *You can be allergic to any food, even foods you have tolerated for years.*

Now that we have laid the foundation for understanding food allergy, we can start to build on this foundation in our quest to understand this allergy. To do this we need to answer a question: Is there only one type of food allergy?

Two Food Allergies

It seems obvious that there is only one program for food allergy. Why should there be two? Two types of food allergy would needlessly complicate the diagnosis and treatment of people who suffer pain and discomfort from foods. It would also lead to confusion and misunderstanding in scientific studies of food allergy if the investigators did not account for both types of food allergy in their studies.

You guessed it—there are two types of food allergy, and they do lead to confusion. Sometimes when you think you suffer from one type of food allergy, you are really being affected by the other. On the other hand, you can suffer from both types at the same time, like a computer programmed to run two different operations at the same time.

Our Programming

Our allergy programming is strange, I admit. That two simultaneous food allergies exist is little appreciated but extremely important in understanding food allergy. The biggest error I see in the reports about food allergy, whether on radio, TV, or in scientific papers, is the failure to appreciate that two types of food allergy cause our symptoms.

Let's make sure you know about the two types of food allergy. To do this, we will first review the symptoms they cause so that we can relate these symptoms to the types of food allergy causing them. We will focus our discussion on:

◇ the symptoms caused by food allergy;
◇ the two separate types of food allergies that cause these symptoms.

The Food Symptoms

Food Allergy Symptoms Appear Quickly or Slowly

We will start by looking at the illnesses food allergies cause, called symptoms. In the section "Overview of Food Allergy and Complications in Diagnosing Food Allergy" above, I described how allergists separate the symptoms of food allergy into two categories: those that appear quickly after eating a food, and those that appear hours later. It is appropriate to review them here.

The quick-appearing symptoms strike within minutes after eating, so we call them "immediate food symptoms." The slow-developing symptoms take hours to appear. They are also appropriately named: "delayed food symptoms." Slowly developing and rapidly developing symptoms sometimes act both similarly and differently.

Rapidly Developing Food Symptoms

If your symptoms appear soon after you eat, you may react like a bee-sensitive person stung by a bee. You may feel mildly annoying symptoms (a little hive, a stuffy nose), or you may be threatened by startling and dangerous symptoms (shock or choking).

Any food can cause immediate food symptoms, including common foods such as milk, wheat, and corn. These common foods seldom cause the dangerous symptoms that threaten your life; other foods, less commonly eaten, do.

Delayed Food Symptoms

Whereas immediate food symptoms act like a bee sting, delayed symptoms act more like influenza. You may suffer painful headaches or abdominal cramps, or you may be overwhelmed by tiredness that saps your energy and confuses your thinking. It may seem as though these flulike symptoms will never stop.

These flulike symptoms are not specific to food allergy. Fibromyalgia causes them; also tension, chronic fatigue syndrome, a cold, or many other illnesses can make you feel as if you have the flu. Because these symptoms are not specific to any illness (unlike the more flamboyant symptoms that proclaim the quick-striking form of food allergy), they confuse the diagnosis, making it harder for you to think of food allergy.

Not only is it difficult to recognize that these ill-defined symptoms are caused by food allergy, it is even more difficult to determine which food to blame. As a result, authors of articles about food allergy tend to cover delayed symptoms poorly and to pay more attention to the easily described and more flamboyant immediate symptoms.

If your knowledge about food allergy depends on such articles, you may be impressed by immediate symptoms and not impressed by delayed reactions. You might even think that few people suffer delayed symptoms and that their symptoms are mild. This is not so; many suffer, and their suffering is great.

We see patient after patient suffering from delayed symptoms to food. Most missed the link between symptoms and food because they thought that food symptoms always strike quickly after eating. It is only when I tell them about delayed symptoms that they start suspecting food allergy.

The Two Types of Food Allergy

If people reacted to foods in only one way—either immediately or delayed—food allergy would be so much easier to understand. Moreover, if only one type of food allergy caused these symptoms, our understanding would be further simplified. However, this is not the case. Food symptoms are caused by two separate food allergies that target two different food components:

1. Type one targets the chemicals in foods.
2. Type two targets the proteins in foods.

Allergy Directed Against the Chemicals in Foods
This is the food allergy I see most frequently in my patients. These foods contain high quantities of the following food chemicals:

<u>M</u>onosodium glutamate

<u>A</u>cidic foods

<u>L</u>ow-calorie sweeteners

Refined <u>S</u>ugar

I use the resulting acronym—MALS—throughout this book to indicate foods containing high quantities of these food chemicals.

The chemicals in our diet. We all like to eat flavorful foods; we load our desserts and candy with refined sugar and our drinks with citrus. We enhance the flavor of our meals with monosodium glutamate (MSG) and enjoy a sweet taste that contributes few calories to our diets—low-calorie sweeteners. Even worse, we consume these chemicals meal after meal, far exceeding our tolerance.

Many of my patients find that when they consume large quantities of these flavor-enhancing chemicals, their head and stomach pains flare. Their throats ache, their noses plug, and their stomachs cramp as they consume their food, so flavorful, sweet, and acidic.

Immediate and delayed symptoms to food chemicals. Symptoms caused by the food chemicals can also appear hours later—and frequently do. For instance, a pizza flavored with MSG at night may provoke a migraine headache the next day (delayed reaction). Alternatively, symptoms may strike quickly after a meal (immediate reaction) if the meal contains so much citrus, sugar, MSG, or low-calorie sweetener that it "overloads" tolerance. Symptoms also strike quickly if previous meals contained such quantities of these chemicals that the present meal, adding its chemicals to the amount in the body, causes a tolerance overload.

Use of the term MALS, which I introduced above, does not imply that the food chemicals listed there are in any way defective or harmful to the nonsensitive person. Each chemical is valuable, produced by competent manufacturers, and useful for people who do not suffer ill effects from them. The "mal" (which in English means undesirable) in MALS applies only to the regrettable symptoms that affect food chemical-sensitive patients.

The name unites four seemingly separate chemicals—monosodium glutamate, acidic foods, low-calorie sweeteners, and refined sugar—into an organized group. These chemicals combine to provoke symptoms. If you eat an MSG-flavored sausage followed by five sugar cookies, your headache came not from MSG or refined sugar individually but from both together. One sensitive person may react most strongly to one of the four chemicals, another person to another chemical. However, even though you must avoid the chemical that bothers you the most, do not focus all your attention on this chemical and ignore the contributions of the other chemicals.

The concept of the food-chemical or MALS food allergy is important to your understanding of food allergy. Among my patients, it is the most important, frequently encountered, and misunderstood of the two food allergies. My patients find that understanding it and eliminating or reducing their consumption of the foods containing high levels of these chemicals relieves many of their symptoms. If you understand it, you will have taken a great step in learning to treat yourself.

Allergy Directed Against the Proteins in Foods

The second type of food allergy is targeted against the proteins in foods.

In company with carbohydrates and fat, all foods contain protein. Among their many uses, they form the backbone of cell walls, enable enzymes to digest food, and transport oxygen around the body.

Certain antibodies that cause allergy act on these proteins. The best known is the IgE antibodies that provoke immediate reactions. They are the same antibodies that direct their actions against proteins in dust, mold, and pollen, and they also find food proteins easy targets.

Certain food proteins more readily draw their attention; for instance, certain proteins of peanut and shrimp strongly attract the IgE antibodies that cause quick-onset choking or hives (a fact unattractive to people suffering from these dangerous reactions).

Just as foods contain protein that can unleash immediate symptoms, they also contain proteins that set off delayed food symptoms. In susceptible people, the milk, wheat, corn, and other food proteins that trip off quick-appearing hives or diarrhea while eating also prompt headaches and abdominal pain that appear the following morning.

I will use the term "classic food allergies" to refer to food-protein allergies in this book.

The Relative Importance of Immediate Versus Delayed Allergy to Food

With its scary and sometimes dangerous symptoms, who can doubt the importance of immediate food symptoms directed against food proteins or food chemicals? In contrast, the consequences of delayed symptoms are uncomfortable but not as dangerous.

Immediate symptoms almost always appear every time an allergic patients eats the offending food. Not so with delayed symptoms. Delayed symptoms do not always follow eating the culprit food.

Certain factors are necessary before they appear, and we discussed them in the section "Overview of Food Allergy and Complications in Diagnosing Food Allergy" above. The factors apply to both food *protein* and food *chemical* allergy. For instance, in both types of food allergy a provoking food might be eaten at a number of meals before the sensitive person eats more of the food than he or she can tolerate.

Once a patient start noticing this delayed pattern, he or she learns to avoid the consequences of eating the food by avoiding eating the same foods daily. The patient also learns to avoid consuming the *amount* of these foods necessary to activate the symptoms. Even when the patient eats an allergy-causing food daily, he or she typically limits consumption to the amount he or she *tolerates*.

If you can determine which foods cause your delayed symptoms, you can learn to use these same procedures to prevent suffering.

Milk is a food many milk-allergic people drink daily but in moderation. Their milk protein allergy shows up on our skin tests, a result greeted with surprise and often disbelief.

When I question patients about the amount of milk in their diet, their answers show that they perhaps subconsciously have learned to restrict their milk intake to the amount they tolerate. Thus they avoid the stuffiness, abdominal pain, or other symptoms of delayed milk allergy, symptoms they would suffer if they consumed milk without restraint.

I realize that you may be confused by these two types of food allergy. Why should you need to absorb all this complicated information? Can it help you understand your food allergy? The answer to both questions is: *If you are unable to separate these two kinds of food allergy in your mind, you will never understand food allergy.* Mary's and Dominic's experiences illustrate this point.

When I question Mary about her food allergy, she states, "Yes, I need to avoid certain foods. If I eat garlic, onions, or eggs, hours later I develop a very painful migraine headache and my stomach hurts. I've learned to avoid them."

Patty's replies to my questions about her son Dominic's food reactions are as follows: "I have to keep chocolate and cheese out of Dominic's diet. If he eats either, he develops severe diarrhea. They also cause terribly painful headaches. And tomatoes and potatoes stuff up his nose."

I then asked, "What about MSG, Patty?"

She replied, "He can't take any MSG. If he does, his face breaks out in a rash that looks like broken blood vessels in his skin."

Mary's allergy to garlic, onions, and eggs is not directed against the food chemicals we have already discussed. It is directed against the protein in these foods. How do we know that they are not directed against their content of food chemicals? Because these foods do not contain excess quantities of acid, sugar, MSG, or low-calorie sweeteners.

In contrast, the foods Dominic must avoid do contain these chemicals: citrus (tomato and potato) and MSG (cheese and tomatoes are naturally high in MSG, and he reacts to MSG used as a flavoring). I'm not sure why he reacts to chocolate; it is such a complex food that several mechanisms may be operating.

In our advice to Mary, we do not need to tell her to avoid foods with high levels of food chemicals—she does not react to them. However, we must tell Dominic to avoid foods with these high levels because he does react to them. These stories show that the correct approach to food allergy treatment depends on whether a person is allergic to food protein, to food chemicals, or to both.

We will begin our study of these food chemicals by following the road I took to discovering their importance. We will focus on these extremely important foods and beverages in the first five sections of chapter 2, examining them one at a time.

MALS Food Chemical Allergy

Citrus: How I Developed a Food Allergy Diet

The events that change our thinking are often peculiar. They leave a lasting impression because they surprise us. They challenge our deeply held beliefs, our concept of order, our most sacred convictions. They turn our view of the world upside down—and stick in our memories.

I remember just such an event, the event that forced me to develop a diet for my patients with food allergy.

It was 1965, and I was a captain in the U.S. Air Force, stationed at Offutt Air Force Base, near Omaha, Nebraska. Medical school and internship completed, I was serving as a general medical officer at the base hospital and clinics. These clinics included pediatrics, internal medicine, ob-gyn, and several other specialty clinics, but there was no allergy clinic because, before I arrived on base, no doctor had been interested in this specialty.

But allergy interested me. Even though I had no allergy training at that time, I knew we could improve the care of the patients with allergy on base if we had a clinic that combined a doctor interested in allergy with nurses trained in allergy. I decided to start this clinic.

I remember one of my first allergy patients, five-year-old Susie. She was dark-haired and adorable, a little sprite with the behavior of a scamp—and skin the texture of course-grained sandpaper. She was suffering from a horrible case of eczema. Her skin looked and felt dry, thick, and red; her constant itching and scratching made her days and nights miserable. Although this aggravating affliction didn't seem to dim her sunny disposition, I pitied her. I could see my pity reflected in the eyes of her father, Bob, who brought her repeatedly to my clinic, hoping I could help.

I tried. I prescribed all the treatments that are supposed to relieve eczema—antihistamines, salves, lotions, avoiding soap, cutting finger-nails short, and wearing gloves at night to reduce damage caused by scratching. My treatment gave her little relief.

Then one day Bob brought Susie in, and she looked great! There had to be a 75-percent improvement in the condition of her skin, and she was no longer red as a lobster.

"I was hoping my treatment would do Susie some good, Bob, and it looks like it finally did," I said, my head swelling with pride. I had conquered Susie's severe eczema! My training and knowledge had finally provided excellent results.

"Well . . . not exactly," said Bob, with an odd look on his face. "None of those treatments you told us to use helped Susie very much. She found her own way of treatment."

"Her own treatment? What is it?" I asked, wondering what she could have possibly discovered.

"Well, when her skin gets really bad, she dumps kitchen cleanser into a bathtub full of water and jumps in. Clears her skin right up."

I was so astonished by his answer, and I am not advocating that you self-treat your eczema with a bath of kitchen cleanser. I have no idea whether kitchen cleanser baths are harmful, so please don't try them. Nevertheless, I wasn't sure what lesson Susie was teaching me. What I did know was that I wanted to help children and adults with eczema, to come up with treatments that would have better results than the pitiful measures I used. Moreover, I knew that before I could unlock the mystery surrounding the diagnosis and treatment of eczema, I would need specialty training in allergy and the practical knowledge I would accumulate over years of treating allergic patients with allergy.

I believe that in cases like Susie's, the body is trying to eliminate the excess acid in the diet by dumping it on the skin, where it contributes to the redness, scaliness, and obnoxious itching characteristic of eczema. Susie was neutralizing the acidity of her skin by soaking in bathwater turned basic by kitchen cleanser. It is a basic law of chemistry that in solution, bases neutralize acids.

Perhaps Susie's kitchen cleanser is a key to learning the cause of this annoying condition. But now I want to talk more about acid in the diet.

Before I could begin to grasp the point of Susie's lesson, another peculiar event occurred, one that was no less surprising. Like my experience with Susie, it made me doubt things I firmly believed to be true, made me discard treatment that should be tried and true, and shook the foundations of what I had been taught about eczema.

It happened years later, after I finished allergy specialty training at the Mayo Clinic and started my practice in St. Paul. It was the fall of 1973, my third year of practice, and increasing numbers of patients were visiting my office. One of these patients was a seven-year-old boy named Mike, a bright child with the solemn manner of a Supreme Court judge and the skin of a torture victim: dry, scaly, and inflamed.

In retrospect, his skin was a lot like Susie's, although it didn't occur to me at the time. If it had, perhaps I might have been prepared for the surprise that awaited me in Mike's case.

Treatment of eczema hadn't improved much since I treated Susie. Mike's dermatologist referred him to me to see if I could find any cause or causes for his rash. I wasn't too hopeful; I found my treatment disappointing and not helped by medical science, which still didn't understand eczema very well.

Mike, his mother, Karen, and I tried various diet and environmental treatments for several months but made no progress; Mike's skin was as dry, scaly, and itchy as the day he first came to my office. Then, on one of Mike's visits, Karen said something that forever changed my thinking on and my treatment of eczema.

"Well, Karen, how's Mike doing?" I asked.

"No change, Dr. Walsh. He's still uncomfortable and itches as much as always."

"That's too bad, Karen. I wish we could be more effective in treating him, but it's hard to do much when we don't even know the cause of eczema." Then I asked, "Karen, have you noticed anything that makes his eczema worse?"

Karen didn't take long to answer. "Yes, I have," she said. "His skin flares up whenever he eats or drinks too much citrus."

Her answer stunned me. Karen impressed me as being a practical and bright woman, not at all likely to be led astray by those old folk tales that blame the acids in foods for illnesses; allergy experts I respected discredited such theories.

Being relatively new to practice, I still hadn't learned to trust my patient, and I still had the inflated ego of the newly trained specialist—I fought against any new ideas that contradicted the teachings I had so laboriously pounded into my head. Thankfully, the realities of medical practice eventually deflate overgrown egos.

Karen's belief that citrus caused Mike's eczema directly contradicted many theories about the cause of eczema. Most allergists agree that eczema is strongly stimulated by allergy, but the idea that patients could be allergic to citrus was preposterous—or so I thought.

Karen's conclusion made no sense to me then for a couple of reasons. First, although people who are allergic to such things as seafood or ragweed react to only tiny parts of the food or the pollen, the part they react to must be at least a certain size. Too small a size and no allergic reaction results. The citrus molecule is too tiny to cause allergy. Like a toy poodle at a greyhound track, it doesn't belong in the race at all.

Second, most of the allergies we know about are directed against proteins; citrus isn't a protein. Not only are they directed against proteins, they also are specifically directed against proteins foreign to the body. But citrus isn't foreign. In fact, citric acid is present in every cell in the body and is one of the compounds involved in energy production.

"Karen, you surprise me," I said. "I thought the fear of food acids was dead and buried. What makes you think citrus bothers Mike?"

"Because he breaks out badly if he eats oranges or grapefruit," she answered, "and he is also miserable if he drinks citrus juices or pop flavored with citrus."

I still wasn't convinced, but I put aside my skepticism for the moment and said, "Okay. Let's get citrus out of his diet and see what happens." I figured it couldn't hurt; I wasn't helping Mike much anyway.

Over the next several weeks, Karen eliminated from Mike's diet all citrus fruits, their juices, and any beverages flavored with citric acid such as sodas and sports drinks. Mike's skin improved remarkably. And not only did his skin improve with citrus eliminated, but also returning these foods and beverages to his diet made his skin red, scaly, and itchy again. Karen was right; citrus—the toy poodle of allergy—was making Mike miserable.

Mike's improvement made me glad I resisted my skepticism. Once I absorbed the implications of citrus-caused allergy, I was eager to try citrus elimination on patients with other allergic illnesses. I tried it on patients with abdominal cramps and diarrhea; many found their cramps diminished and the diarrhea less. I tried it on patients with hives; many suffered fewer hives. I tried it on patients with stuffed noses; in many, the stuffiness subsided. Some asthmatic patients wheezed less. Even many of my hay fever patients responded to elimination; if they avoided citrus, their pollen reactions eased up. I was impressed and excited.

Obviously citrus bothered many of my patients and was one of the factors causing their allergic illnesses. But why? I can't say for sure, but I suspect it may have something to do with the human body's ability to adapt to change.

Even though each of our cells contains a small amount of citric acid, our bodies may be unable to handle large amounts of this acid. This is probably because these large quantities of citrus are a recent addition to our diets, and our digestive, metabolic, and elimination processes haven't yet adjusted to dealing with excess citrus.

I know this may seem surprising; experts believe citrus cultivation started in China four thousand years ago. Four thousand years should be long enough to adapt to a new diet with excess citrus. But when you consider that we digest, metabolize, and eliminate our food in the same way as our primitive ancestors who dodged the footsteps of dinosaurs eighty million years ago, four thousand years is but a blink of evolution's eye—not enough time to evolve an innovative ability to handle a new diet.

Our modern food production system is partly responsible for us consuming huge amounts of citrus and other food acids; just check the ingredients on the canned and packaged foods in your pantry to see how many contain acidic ingredients. And our present generation's eating habits have increased the incidence of acidic foods in our diet—grapefruit juice in the morning, tomato slices in our sandwiches and an orange at noon, potatoes and strawberry ice cream at dinner, and grapes as a late-night snack.

This list emphasizes another surprising point: all of the foods mentioned are acidic. I didn't know foods such as strawberries and potatoes were acidic when Karen told me about Mike's reaction to citric acid, but I discovered that they were when I learned about certain inconsistencies that arose in treating other patients. Why did Dick's migraines strike when he drank apple juice, which contains mostly malic acid? Why did Alice's diarrhea flare up after eating candy with fumaric acid? Obviously, acids other then citric acid were causing allergic distress.

Acids in Our Diet

Citric, fumaric, malic acids—the names are familiar. Each of them participates in the Krebs cycle, the process that changes food to energy, the process we will examine in chapter 3 under the section "Why We Are Allergic to Foods." As energy is released, the acids are torn apart, which changes one acid into another. Citric acid changes to succinic acid, succinic acid to fumaric, fumaric to malic, then—after a little repair to the tattered acid—back to citric acid again.

Of all the acids we find in our diet, citric acid is most important because it is the one most widely used. Its pleasant, sour, fruity taste makes it a perfect flavoring agent for beverages, candy, pies, and many other treats. Manufacturers use it in the pharmaceutical industry, usually in amounts too small to cause symptoms—except in one case I remember well.

I met Jean, a seventy-six-year-old retired kindergarten teacher, when her internist asked me to examine her in the hospital just after her bowel surgery. Prior to surgery, she was given medicine to clear the stools out of her colon. The medicine worked too well—she suffered a frightful case of diarrhea. Not only did she suffer diarrhea, but also her blood pressure plunged so low that she almost went into shock, and it took days for her to recover from this overpowering reaction.

Her internist and surgeon were stumped: "All we gave her was a dose of harmless magnesium citrate," they told me. Citrate is another name for citrus, and after battling the diarrhea that citrus caused some of my patients, what happened stumped me not at all. I did not share their belief that, in Jean's case, citrate was harmless. However, the experience did help me realize that other doctors had no concept of the illness that could be caused in certain allergic patients by large doses of citrus.

Other Acids

Malic acid, the major acid in apples, is second in importance and frequency of use to citric acid. Much like citric acid, it has a pleasant, sour, fruity taste and is used to flavor foods and beverages and in pharmaceutical products.

Fumaric and succinic acids are seldom used in foods or beverages, although I have noticed fumaric in some candies, and both are used in drug manufacturing, where the levels seem too low to bother my patients. The names of these acids can sometimes be confusing. For all practical purposes, citrate and citric acid are the same, as are succinate and succinic acid, fumarate and fumaric acid, and malate and malic acid.

The more I investigate acidic foods and their effect on my patients, the more complicated it becomes—multiple foods, multiple illnesses, multiple acids. Every time I think I finally understand it all, new information surfaces. It's like carrying a sheet of four-by-eight-foot plywood on a windy day—every time you take four steps forward, a new gust comes along and blows you three steps backward.

For instance, just as I was congratulating myself on knowing all the acids that made my patients sick, I found a new one. Tartaric acid or tartrate, the main acid in grapes, grape juice, grape-flavored drinks, wine, cognac and brandy, causes particularly severe reactions in some of my patients, including headaches, hives, eczema, cramps, diarrhea, and many others. That discovery taught me to be constantly on the lookout.

And Even More Acidic Foods

I am glad I continued to search. I found a number of good references that helped this search. Through them I learned that many foods other than oranges, lemons, limes, and grapefruit are acidic. Tomatoes, berries, and cherries are acidic, often more so than the citrus fruits.

I was shocked to find that the ordinary potato is acidic. It wasn't even on my list of suspects. The potato is related to the tomato; the leaves look like tomato leaves, and the seed looks like a tiny green tomato. I understand that both came from the same plant, with the potato growing below ground and the tomato up on the plant in the sunlight.

That helps explain why many of my patients suffer if they eat potatoes. I found that potatoes cause the same symptoms as tomatoes if eaten in excess of my patients' tolerance level, a level that is sometimes very low.

The Importance of Acid in the Diet

When I first began telling my patients that they might be allergic to acidic foods, they were overwhelmed by the complexity of changing their eating habits. I couldn't blame them for looking at me with evident confusion and asking, "What should I avoid?" A mumbled response that they should avoid all acidic foods didn't ease their confusion one bit. They needed to have the diet written down so they could understand it, so I began to do so. I revised it when my staff and I learned more, and I revised it again and again and again. And that's how the diet has evolved to where it is today.

I believe that discovering the role of acidic foods in many of my patients' symptoms is a significant advance in the diagnosis and treatment of allergic illness. However, lest you think I praise myself for this discovery, let me assure you I had not meant to give you this impression. My patients discovered this allergy, not I.

I know that you must be wondering where all these acid foods are in the diet. After we examine the other food chemicals you must watch, I will list these chemicals in the elimination diet that explores this food allergy.

I wish that allergy to food acids did not exist. For those allergic patients who eat acidic foods without distress, enjoy them. They are excellent foods and beverages packed with refreshing taste and great nutrition.

For those who must suffer from this most unkind allergy, a delicious part of the diet becomes a source of pain and discomfort. If you react to acidic foods, I regret that you must limit the acid in your diet to the amount you tolerate without symptoms. I also must avoid acidic foods; they bring me heartburn and abdominal, ulcerlike pain.

My patients' dietary restrictions extend beyond the delicious acidic foods and beverages enjoyed by the nonallergic person. Other equally delicious foods and beverages must be avoided by many of our unfortunate patients. One of these, the delightfully effective flavoring agent monosodium glutamate (MSG), is the subject of the next section.

Monosodium Glutamate (Alias MSG)

A doctor should strive to nurture and protect his or her patients and to improve their precious health. This ancient and honorable mission imposes a heavy burden of responsibility on doctors and other health care professions, an obligation to shield our patients and the community at large from the dangers we perceive. I believe all medical care professionals feel this obligation. I know that I do.

For me, nothing heightens this sense of obligation more than my experiences with monosodium glutamate, a food chemical my staff and I try our darnedest to reduce or eliminate from our patients' diets if they react to it. I don't mean to be an alarmist, but the frequency with which I encounter the effects of MSG in my patients' illnesses and its presence in so many of the foods we eat worry me greatly. Perhaps when I tell you about some of my experiences with this dietary chemical, you will understand and perhaps share my concern. I will start with how I discovered that it bothered patients.

I was delighted with the improvement in my patients' symptoms when I started to understand the significance of the acidic foods and beverages. When patients reduced or eliminated them, headaches decreased, cramps and diarrhea slowed, hives sprouted less, eczema itched less, noses unblocked, and wheezing declined.

However, I was also perplexed. Although my patients' symptoms diminished, they did not disappear. In fact, they still suffered plenty of headaches, hives, diarrhea, and all the other maladies to which the allergic person is prey. I suspected that foods caused these symptoms, and I needed to expand my knowledge of food allergy to find these additional culprits. Where were these foods? What was missing?

What was missing was my willingness to listen to my patients. I hadn't yet learned an important lesson of medical practice: the people who know the most about the cause of patients' illnesses are the patients themselves.

Like a choir whose distant voice I heard but poorly, they continued to tell me about other ingredients in the diet that made them ill. But I did not listen closely enough. They told me about foods that were not acidic but that caused pain and discomfort. I didn't hear them. I finally heard them when a friend who suffered with cluster headaches added his voice.

Although the many allergy symptoms bestowed on me include sinus headaches, I count myself fortunate in never suffering from cluster headaches, one of the most painful of human afflictions. In cluster headaches, the nerves of the face and scalp ache with overwhelming intensity. John had such headaches. He had tried every known medical treatment he could find. When one of these painful headaches struck, he found relief only from inhaling pure oxygen.

I tried treating him with allergy injections and eliminating acid from his diet. It helped, but he still had unexplained headaches. Then one day John complained of a particularly brutal headache, which prompted the following discussion:

"Bill, I had a horrible headache last night."

"How did it happen, John?" I asked.

"I was at a meeting where they served snacks," he said. "I wasn't hungry, but you know how you munch just to keep your hands busy. I ate some sausages that were excellent. On the way home I got hit with a headache so painful I had trouble seeing where I was driving. I hurt so badly I wasn't able to break it with oxygen." He sighed. "The pain kept me up all night."

"John, did you eat anything else?" I asked.

"No."

"Did you drink anything?" I tried again.

"Just water," he replied, shrugging his shoulders.

John looked pale and worn out after his night of dreadful pain. I was also curious: Was there some clue to John's pain in that sausage? We tracked down the ingredients in the sausage and found that they included monosodium glutamate—MSG.

Then I remembered that patients had often told me monosodium glutamate caused them headaches or diarrhea. But I had dismissed their observations, thinking it wasn't the MSG but their own imagination that was at fault. After all, studies by medical scientists showed that monosodium glutamate rarely caused illness. But I was to find that the medical scientists and I were wrong and my patients were right.

What Is Monosodium Glutamate?

For those who aren't very familiar with MSG, a short description should help. It's not strange or unnatural; it's found in all your body proteins. Moreover, it's not synthetic. Every plant and animal manufactures it.

MSG makes up a major part of proteins, which are composed of individual amino acids, much as a chain is made of individual links. Glutamic acid is one of the amino acid links in protein; there it composes 10 to 40 percent of the proteins—a lot. When glutamic acid is freed from the protein chain, it is soluble (floats) in water or body fluids, where it meets a sodium molecule (part of table salt) that floats with it. Hence the name monosodium (one salt) glutamate (free glutamic acid)—shortened to MSG.

How does it trouble my patients? I believe that while glutamic acid remains firmly anchored in intact protein, it causes no harm. It is firmly held captive, released slowly only when the body is ready for it, slowly enough so the body can handle it at its own pace.

In all foods, some of the glutamic acid is freed from protein. Since it is not bound to protein, this free glutamic acid, called MSG, is probably absorbed very quickly. If the amount of MSG is small, its impact is also small or nonexistent. However, if the amount is large, its fast release and adsorption can overwhelm the body's metabolism. When the body's metabolism fails to handle it, troubles erupt.

Illnesses Caused by MSG

MSG causes illnesses that vary from patient to patient. Debbie, a thirty-one-year-old labor and delivery nurse, told me about her reactions. Our conversation began something like this:

"How are the allergy shots treating you, Debbie?"

"They help a lot as long as I get them every two weeks," she said. "If I let them go beyond two weeks, my nose gets stuffy and I feel tired."

"How about your diet? Any foods give you trouble?" I asked.

"I have to avoid the acidic foods or my cold sores flare up. As a nurse I look horrible with a big cold sore on my lips, and my patients think I have some terrible disease."

"Any trouble with MSG, Debbie?"

"I have to avoid it completely. I read every label, so it's not too hard to avoid in my own cooking, but sometimes I'll eat it at a restaurant or at dinner at a friend's house. I'm too embarrassed to ask them if they use MSG," she admitted. "They'd probably think I'm a kook."

"I know what you mean about eating at a friend's house," I sympathized. "What does MSG do to you?"

"It's really bad, Dr. Walsh. First, I develop a terrible thirst. Then I get puffy and bloated and my clothes get really tight, and I can't wear a belt because my stomach hurts. I get hyper, and for several nights I can't sleep. And all my joints ache."

Debbie's reaction to MSG is not rare, unusual, or a figment of her imagination. Many other patients complain of similar symptoms. I also share them. I always ask at a restaurant if they use MSG and try to choose foods that aren't likely to contain it, but sometimes I get it anyway. My good friends know not to use it in meals they prepare for me, but I feel strange questioning the hostess about MSG if I don't know her well. Like Debbie, I don't want to sound like a kook.

When I get MSG, it gets me. Hours later, a huge thirst develops; I feel puffy and bloated—my hands swell so much they feel like sausages. My belt tightens around my waist and the numbers on my bathroom scale creep upward, showing five extra pounds that stay for about three days, then drop off. (The swelling I have described is similar to the fluid accumulation that afflicts many people. I often wonder how many of them could trade their water pills for a better treatment—a diet change.)

After eating foods with MSG, I sleep miserably for about three nights until the bloating stops and the scale drops. My stomach churns with acid, and like Debbie, I have nagging joint pain; my bad knee swells and aches for three days.

I see these same symptoms in many patients: puffiness, bloating, abdominal discomfort, joint achiness, irritability, and insomnia. The list of symptoms goes on and on. Other patients suffer different symptoms; their asthma worsens, their stuffy noses drip and their hearing drops, hives flare, and eczema itches more. For those who suffer headaches, their sinus pressure/pain increases measurably; migraine sufferers experience nearly unbearable surges of pain. (Many of my numerous patients with frequent headaches tolerate MSG poorly.)

My patients who experience pain and discomfort from MSG seldom encounter life-threatening symptoms, but the pain and discomfort are so hurtful that many must avoid it as they would avoid playing with a loaded gun. However, not all people react to MSG. The subject of MSG must be approached with a sense of proportion. It does not cause all allergic symptoms, although it causes many. Allergy is too complex a matter to attribute all symptoms to a single food or food chemical; logic tells us that numerous causes spawn these numerous illnesses.

However, it is important to recognize that this dietary component often provokes uncomfortable, painful, and even dangerous illness. I suspect that many people with allergies have a susceptibility to MSG.

Where Is MSG Found?

When I began looking for acidic foods, I foolishly thought they would be easy to find. Instead, I found there were many sources and types of acids, and they could crop up in the strangest places. It was the same with MSG.

At first I thought, What could be easier? Read your labels, stop using spices that contain MSG, and when you dine out, tell the server you want your meal prepared without it. How smart of me to solve the problem. Unfortunately, I found out it's not that easy.

When you tell the server not to use MSG, you may get a confused expression and the response "What's MSG?" Or, even worse, an attempt to appease you by assuring you, "We don't use MSG in our cooking," and then unwittingly bringing you a meal loaded with it. How often that's happened to me.

Fortunately, restaurants are becoming more knowledgeable about MSG and the foods that contain it. Unfortunately, they are not always aware of the difficulty of identifying all the foods containing it.

You will also find it difficult to identify foods containing MSG. Reading labels is the right thing to do, but you must read every label. MSG enhances the flavor of many dishes, especially meat, breading, and soups, but you can find it anywhere in the diet. Always read every label.

MSG is also difficult to identify because it is hidden within other food additives or is the result of food processing, as we shall see.

Hydrolyzed Vegetable Protein

MSG must be mentioned on every label where it is used in its pure form. However, if food manufacturers add it as an ingredient that is part of another ingredient, such as hydrolyzed vegetable protein, they do not need to list MSG on the label, even if a large amount of MSG is involved.

I am sure the food manufacturer means no harm by not mentioning its presence. After all, MSG is on the FDA's "generally recognized as safe" (or GRAS) list of flavoring agents. However, for my patients, not listing MSG on the label has the same effect as if the manufacturer were hiding it in a sneaky and underhanded way.

Hydrolyzed vegetable protein is simply vegetable protein that is broken down (hydrolyzed) into its constituent amino acids. Since protein, including vegetable protein, is 10 to 40 percent glutamic acid, hydrolyzed vegetable protein contains between 10 to 40 percent monosodium glutamate. Remember, protein-bound glutamic acid doesn't hurt my patients. The harm comes when the glutamic acid is released from the protein and becomes the free and rapidly absorbed monosodium glutamate.

I once went to a food show where a food manufacturer was proudly advertising its "MSG-free" products. When I read the label on the soups it was promoting, I noticed that each soup contained hydrolyzed vegetable protein. I'm afraid I made a spectacle of myself berating the poor salespeople about their suspicious advertising practices and telling them that if my patients ate their soups, they would become exceedingly ill.

I made no headway by berating the unfortunate salespeople; they weren't the ones who formulated the soup. But you can make a difference if you see a product with hydrolyzed vegetable protein that is not labeled as containing MSG. Complain to the store manager—he or she doesn't want to lose you as a customer. When the store manager complains to the food companies, perhaps they will listen and admit to using MSG in their product. A letter to the manufacturer could be equally effective.

By the way, when dining in a restaurant, ask for a simple meat, fish, or poultry dish—no sauces—and ask that no spices be put on it. Then hope for the best. Also, hope that the food did not arrive in the restaurant preseasoned with MSG.

Fermentation and MSG

I thought I had discovered all the sources of MSG when I found it in spices and in hydrolyzed vegetable protein. I was wrong. Some of my patients told me they suffered MSG-like symptoms when they ate cheese. That sounded strange because cheese is made of milk, and milk doesn't have high levels of MSG. I searched for and found reference books on MSG that explained the mystery.

Milk protein is 20 percent glutamic acid, most of it firmly bound to protein so the body can slowly digest and absorb it. However, in the cheese-making process, the milk protein is fermented, breaking apart the protein and releasing MSG. It seems that the more aged the cheese, the more milk protein is digested, and the more MSG is released. In fact, much to my distress, as I like cheese, some of the foods highest in MSG are varieties of aged cheese. What a shame!

Any fermentation process, in fact, will break down protein, releasing MSG. Soy sauce, a frequently used fermented product, contains MSG, and my patients find they must avoid it or suffer severe consequences. Fermentation may also be one of the reasons why so many patients with allergies can't tolerate alcoholic drinks. Many of my food-sensitive patients react severely to wine, probably because of the combination of citric and tartaric acids along with the fermentation-released MSG.

Yet another way to manufacture MSG is to allow yeast to digest itself and, in doing so, cause the digestive enzymes to release glutamic acid from the yeast protein, producing MSG. This product is called autolyzed (self-digested) yeast or yeast extract.

The moral of the story? Beware of all fermented preparations.

High Free-Glutamate Levels in Certain Foods

I made another discovery while reading about MSG. Certain foods naturally contain high levels of free glutamic acid or MSG, and patients with sensitivity to MSG must approach them cautiously. They include peas, corn, mushrooms, and tomatoes.

Eating peas and corn may be acceptable for many MSG-sensitive people. I suspect a good boiling will remove much of the water-soluble MSG, especially in corn removed from the cob before boiling. Cutting it from the cob opens each kernel, exposing it to the boiling water.

I have personal experience with corn intolerance. I consider corn on the cob to be one of the foods of the gods; I love its sweet, succulent taste, especially when drenched in butter. However, it doesn't love me. Corn on the cob gives me all the symptoms I get from eating MSG—bloating, acid stomach, insomnia—but I tolerate and enjoy corn cut from the cob and boiled until it is soft. A surprising number of my patients share my experience.

Mushrooms and tomatoes cannot be processed in the same way. In fact, removing the MSG from these foods would probably make them so bland we wouldn't care to have them in our diet. The combination of MSG and acid in tomatoes must be the reason why they are so highly prized as flavoring in our foods. Its citrus and MSG must also be the reason why many of my patients react to tomatoes. The same may be true of potatoes. Converting tomatoes to various sauces and purées concentrates its MSG and increases its concentration.

Watch out for peas, corn, mushrooms, and tomatoes! If they cause you no distress, eat them and enjoy their fine taste. If they cause you distress, consume them with care.

A Letter from the Food and Drug Administration

I wondered how the Food and Drug Administration (FDA) regarded MSG, so I obtained its report on the Internet called the FDA Backgrounder, dated August 31, 1995, and titled "FDA and Monosodium Glutamate (MSG)." The following items from this report and a previous report, dated October 1991 and titled "Monosodium Glutamate (MSG)," help us understand MSG.

The reports review the use of MSG as a flavor enhancer for the past two thousand years. The 1991 Backgrounder stated that it was first used "in the form of a broth made with the types of seaweed known as sea tangle." It is manufactured today using starch and sugar fermentation and is called MSG or calcium or potassium glutamate. MSG is useful as a flavor enhancer in its free amino acid form, and "part of the flavor-enhancing effect of tomatoes, certain cheeses, and fermented or hydrolyzed protein products is due to the presence of free glutamate."

The FDA has conducted and continues to conduct extensive evaluations of the safety of MSG. "Until evaluation is complete, MSG remains on the GRAS list with a requirement that it must be identified as 'monosodium glutamate' on the ingredient label of any food to which it is added."

The Backgrounder from 1995 discusses the FDA's concern about the use of MSG in foods where the presence of this product is not noted on the label—for instance, when hydrolyzed vegetable protein is used without noting that it contains MSG. The FDA states, ". . . FDA considers foods whose labels say 'No MSG' or 'No Added MSG' to be misleading if the food contains ingredients that are sources of free glutamates, such as hydrolyzed protein."

In 1993 the FDA proposed adding the phrase "(contains glutamate)" to the common or usual name for the hydrolysates that contain substantial amounts of glutamate. For example, the label would state "hydrolyzed soy protein (contains glutamate)."

Let's hope this proposal eventually becomes law and that MSG is more clearly identified on the labels of the foods we buy. For those who must avoid it, this labeling will be a tremendous help. It would also be a tremendous help to label the amount of MSG present in a food, as many of my patients can tolerate only certain amounts of MSG.

A Helpful List

Included in the 1991 Backgrounder from the FDA was a helpful (although according to their disclaimer not comprehensive) list that I am reproducing below in its entirety:

A. The following ingredients contain glutamates (including MSG), with the percentages of glutamate content indicated in the parentheses:

> Monosodium glutamate (99 percent)
> Hydrolyzed vegetable protein, hydrolyzed plant protein, or protein hydrolysate (5 to 20 percent)
> Autolyzed yeast extract (5 to 12 percent)
> Sodium or calcium caseinate (about 1 percent)
> Aged cheese, such as Parmesan and Roquefort (about 1 percent)

B. The following ingredients may contain glutamates (including MSG), but the amounts of glutamate content can range from very small to significant, depending on their formulations:

    Flavorings
    Natural flavorings
    Natural beef flavoring
    Natural chicken flavoring
    Natural pork flavoring

C. The following ingredients may contain glutamates (including MSG), but the amounts of glutamate content can range from very small to significant, depending on their manufacturing conditions:
    Bouillon
    Broth
    Stock
    Tomato paste
    Textured protein
    Whey protein
    Dried yeasts, Torula yeast, and yeast nutrients

You may be tempted to decide that flavorings containing pure monosodium glutamate must be avoided because they contain 99 percent MSG but that autolyzed yeast extract (5 to 12 percent MSG) or aged cheese (1 percent MSG) can be eaten with safety. This is not so.

What matters is how much MSG ends up in your stomach. If the food manufacturer added a large amount of autolyzed yeast extract to the food, the content of yeast-derived MSG may be much higher in the food than if a small amount of pure MSG were added. For those who suffer from MSG, it is enough to know that an MSG-containing flavoring was added—we must avoid it. Don't buy the food. Don't eat it.

This report also shows that only a small amount of MSG is needed to flavor food. I am amazed that such a small quantity of MSG—1 percent in the case of aged cheese—can cause patients so much distress.

The impact of MSG on some patients is enormous; it causes severe illness to those who react to it. Its constant presence in our diet makes it difficult to avoid, but the misery it causes patients who react to it makes avoidance imperative.

I find it hard to believe that my patients are the only allergic people affected by MSG. The odds are that many people who are not my patients are susceptible, and I am concerned that they are unaware of their sensitivity. Being unaware, they have no way of knowing that they should avoid this chemical.

I also worry that MSG may be causing more harm than the allergic symptoms I see in my practice. There is good evidence MSG is excitotoxic—that is, it excites and damages nerves. The implications of this excitotoxicity are profound, and we will examine them as we discuss other dietary chemicals that my patients must avoid.

The Social Issues Committee of the Society for Neuroscience discussed effect on nerves at some length, as reported in the January 1990 issue of *Science* magazine. They note that "excitotoxic compounds mimicking glutamate's actions have been found to occur naturally in some foods at levels high enough to cause brain damage when eaten. Excitotoxins have been linked to a diet-related spastic disease in parts of Africa and Asia, to a neurodegenerative disease on Guam, and to a shellfish poisoning incident in Canada that causes a form of memory loss resembling Alzheimer's disease."

They also point out that a buildup of glutamate in the brain may be a cause of brain damage in stroke, hypoglycemia, trauma, and seizure. In addition, some researchers propose that the nerve degeneration in Parkinson's and Alzheimer's diseases may be at least partially due to "glutamate metabolism gone awry." These diseases linked to excitotoxic amino acids caused the committee members to worry about the use of MSG in the foods we eat.

The concern raised by the findings of this committee may be heightened by a study reported in May 1992 in the highly respected *New England Journal of Medicine*. The authors studied amyotrophic lateral sclerosis, a chronic disease characterized by progressive muscle weakness and wasting, and finally death. Better known as Lou Gehrig's disease, it kills one person in every thousand. They found a defect in the nerve cell's handling of glutamic acid that may allow this excitotoxic amino acid to accumulate around the nerve in high enough quantities to damage and ultimately kill it. I do not know if this is a cause of the disease, but I worry about the possibility and wonder if a similar though less severe reaction may occur in people without this disease.

In its 1995 Backgrounder, the FDA acknowledges the tie between MSG and diseases of the nervous system. "Studies show that the body uses glutamate, an amino acid, as a nerve impulse transmitter in the brain and that there are glutamate-responsive tissues in other parts of the body as well. Abnormal function of the glutamate receptors have been linked with certain neurological diseases, such as Alzheimer's disease and Huntington's chorea. Injections of glutamate have resulted in damage to nerve cells in the brain."

What a crazy world where the federal government closely regulates drugs, is in the process of closely regulating alcohol, tobacco, and fat, and gingerly tiptoes around the regulation, even the identification, of an unsupervised, widely used dietary neurotoxin.

What Does All of This Mean?

Perhaps, some critics would say, it is nothing more than another set of far-fetched claims by experts whose imaginations are working overtime, experts foolish enough to think a flavoring agent could cause harm when it is so safe it can be fed to babies.

I do not agree with these critics. I believe it may be one of those keys I talked about in chapter 1, one that will open the door to further research that will one day prove illnesses caused by excitotoxic amino acids to be far more common than we suspect today.

Finally, it may mean that those who feel sorry for my patients because they cannot eat MSG-containing foods are wrong. As they dine with their families on a meal of delicious turkey injected with hydrolyzed vegetable protein, perhaps a discomforting thought should stray across their minds. Perhaps ultimately they will find that the people to pity are themselves, who may for years have eaten an amino acid that is neurotoxic.

Our exploration of the field of food allergy requires us to branch off onto two other paths; in the next section we will follow the first one—the path leading to low-calorie sweetener allergy. As we shall discover, it is an important path to follow.

Low-Calorie Sweeteners

Of all the dietary chemicals we ask our patients to avoid, I have the least experience with low-calorie food and beverage sweeteners.

This is not the case with other dietary chemicals. Because my patients with MSG and citrus sensitivity happen onto MSG-laced meals or devour too much acidic food on many occasions, I frequently hear stories of pain and suffering from their use. These stories keep problems caused by acidic foods and MSG fresh in my mind.

Not so with low-calorie sweeteners. They are easy to identify, and our patients seem to have an innate suspicion of them. Most patients eliminate them from their diet immediately and never return to using them. Therefore, they do not experience the symptoms they might cause, symptoms that would clarify my understanding of low-calorie sweeteners.

My best glimpse of these symptoms comes when new patients who have been using high quantities of low-calorie sweeteners stop their use and observe the symptoms that lessen or disappear. I also see their effects in those patients who continue using them while following the rest of our dietary advice.

The symptoms they mention include those we see in MSG-sensitive patients: headache, bloating, irritability, difficulty in concentrating, hives, eczema, abdominal cramps, diarrhea, nasal blockage, wheezing, joint and muscle aches, and many others. Eliminating low-calorie sweeteners seems to eliminate those symptoms.

Although I have less experience with low-calorie sweeteners than with other components of the diet, based on my day-to-day practice, I believe they cause illnesses. I also believe that my patients must avoid them. Proceeding on the assumption that this is correct, let's examine them further.

What Are the Low-Calorie Sweeteners?

The two most widely used sweeteners are saccharin and aspartame. Saccharin is not frequently used by my patients; however, a number do use aspartame, which sweetens a multitude of foods and beverages, including breakfast cereal, chewing gum, cocoa, instant iced tea, and alcoholic beverage mixes. Equal, a granulated sugar substitute, is made of aspartame. NutraSweet—aspartame again—sweetens many carbonated and noncarbonated beverages.

Aspartame is made of aspartic acid and phenylalanine, two of the amino acids that the body uses to make protein. (We already know that the glutamic acid that makes MSG is another of these amino acids.) Although they are bound together in the aspartame molecule, the amino acids seem to break apart rapidly in digestion, releasing them both and allowing rapid absorption into the body, as in the case of MSG.

Aspartic Acid in Manufactured Sweeteners

Fortunately, we encounter aspartic acid less frequently in our diet than acidic foods and MSG. As with MSG, it is not the aspartic acid locked into protein that concerns us. The intact protein slows digestion by the need to break the amino acid free of the protein, retarding the rate of absorption. Slower absorption allows the body to handle the aspartic acid load at a pace that it finds comfortable.

The aspartic acid in our diet that concerns us is that which can be absorbed quickly. The most familiar source is the low-calorie sweetener I mentioned, aspartame, sold under the brand names NutraSweet and Equal. It is easy to avoid, and my patients generally abstain from its use.

Aspartic Acid in Unprocessed Foods

Free aspartic acid is also found naturally in unprocessed foods. Grapefruit has appreciable quantities, grapefruit juice even more. Oranges and their juice, strawberries, nectarines, plums, and prunes (especially dried prunes) also contain considerable amounts of aspartic acid. In addition, these fruits contain significant amounts of citric acids, making them doubly distressing for my patients who react to consuming excess aspartic and citric acids.

My patients tolerate peaches, perhaps because they contain only half the citric and malic acid of oranges, but peach juice concentrates both of those acids as well as the aspartic acid of the fruit. This combination of citric and malic acid plus aspartic acid is a good illustration of why many of my patients find that they have to avoid any fruit juice. Tomato juice, which concentrates the tomato's low aspartic acid content plus its high glutamic acid content, is another good illustration.

Low-calorie sweeteners came into my elimination diet as an unwelcome guest. They made the diet more complicated for my unfortunate patients and gave them yet other dietary chemicals to avoid.

However, their presence, especially as they focused my attention on aspartic acid, provided a key to understanding both the diet and allergic disorders. It drew my attention to the role of the Krebs cycle in causing allergic illness, most likely through toxic or stimulating effects on the nerves.

Allergic illness due to dietary chemicals may result at least partially from harmful effects on these damaged or irritated nerves. We will explore this possibility next.

Glutamic and Aspartic Acids

I knew about aspartic acid, part of the low-calorie-sweetener molecule, but I didn't pay much attention to it until it was mentioned in some material that I was reading to learn more about the glutamic acid element of MSG. I found a number of reference books on glutamic acid, as well as symposium papers and textbooks written by scientists who study it. I confess that I was unable to thoroughly understand what they were saying. Most of the papers were directed at scientists who are familiar with the jargon of the field and not at the occasional allergist who might try to read them.

Even though I did not fully comprehend those references, I understood certain facts that pointed to an explanation of my patients' unfortunate reactions to the dietary chemicals we ask them to avoid. Although the following is speculative, I believe it is true. I also believe you deserve to know these facts. They explain why I believe that my sensitive patients must avoid these chemicals.

Excitotoxic Amino Acids

In the reference works I studied, aspartic acid and glutamic acid (MSG) were mentioned together because their actions are similar. In the section on MSG I described some of the evidence that indicates MSG may cause illness. I also reviewed the concerns expressed by some scientists who question its safety as a flavoring agent in our diet.

Both glutamic and aspartic acids are included in the category of excitotoxic amino acids because of their ability to excite or stimulate nerve cells of animals, including humans. This nerve stimulation may lead to nerve degeneration. In excess quantities, especially in the young animal, both glutamic and aspartic acids are also neurotoxic, or poisonous, to nerves. That's worrisome!

Of course, our ordinary diet does not subject us to the excessive quantity of these amino acids used in the studies that showed nerve damage in animals. Nor do we share the susceptibility of the fetal or newborn animal to these injurious effects.

But what if there were a population of humans who suffered nerve degeneration from long-term, low-dose exposure in the diet? Perhaps the threat would be even greater if other diet chemicals—such as food acids—potentiated or aided in this damage. What if we called this population of people allergic patients?

I know this theory probably sounds a little preposterous, but there is some evidence to support it. First of all, nerves are involved in some allergic illnesses. The following are examples of these illnesses in which nerve injury or degeneration is a factor.

Cold sores, those recurring and unattractive ulcers of the lips, are caused by a virus infection of the nerves of the lips. My patients find that if they closely follow our dietary recommendations, especially if they drastically reduce their intake of acidic foods, their cold sores hurt them less and seem to swell less. I know this firsthand because I get cold sores myself. Even if I watch my diet, I still get cold sores, but they are not as large or as painful if I avoid the food chemicals.

My experience and the experience of my patients indicate that dietary avoidance does not cure cold sores, but it stops the spread of the lip rash. Evidently the chemicals in foods, especially acids, further injure the virus-damaged nerve that is causing the ulcer, indicating that they are neurotoxic to that nerve.

Eczema

Another piece of evidence that I find impressive arises from studies on eczema, the irritating skin disease that is marked by constant severe itching. Biopsies of eczema skin show damage to the nerves that supply the skin. Many regard this evidence of nerve degeneration to be not a cause but a consequence of eczema. But what if it is actually the cause? What if the skin nerves were injured by the dietary chemicals that cause my patients so much trouble, and the damaged nerves sent impulses of itchiness to the brain? What if this itching sensation caused my patients to scratch their skin so hard and so frequently that it became dry, red, swollen, and even cracked? Perhaps this is how eczema develops. I believe that this hypothesis is true.

If this is so, then the treatment, of course, is to remove neurotoxic chemicals from the diet as much as possible. By now you shouldn't be surprised when I tell you that removing acidic foods, MSG, and aspartic acid from the diet reduces the itchiness and eczema of many of my patients, allowing their skin to improve markedly.

Nerve Damage in Allergic Illness

I could give you many more examples of allergic illnesses, including such common afflictions as headaches, asthma, and hives, that give evidence of nerve degeneration or excitation. In each case the evidence is intriguing and, I'd like to think, persuasive. Suffice it to say that I believe that these examples support my theory that dietary chemicals, including food acids, may contribute to nerve damage.

This theory is especially significant because it can be a key to explaining a great deal about food allergy. For instance, why does food allergy affect so many areas of the body? Is it through the nerves? It also can help explain how these food chemicals cause unrelated illnesses such as diarrhea and hives in the same patient, again through their connection to nerves.

Relationships Among Allergic Symptoms

It might not seem that allergic symptoms that affect different areas of the body are related, but they are. In the explanation I just gave you, food chemicals do not need to attack the colon and the skin directly, just the nerves supplying the colon and the skin. The irritated nerves throw the colon into spasm, causing abdominal pain and diarrhea. In the skin, this same damage will fire off the motor nerves, dilating blood vessels (making the skin red) and allowing fluid to leak from these dilated vessels (causing the hive bump). The damaged sensory nerves in the dilated blood vessels send itch sensations to the brain. That's why the same allergic reaction can deliver abdominal pain and diarrhea as well as red, itchy, and bumpy skin.

Nerve damage caused by dietary chemicals also can explain other allergic illnesses. In migraine headaches, the stimulated nerves controlling the blood vessels of the head contract and then dilate these vessels, affecting the surrounding nerve fibers that carry the sensation of pain to the brain. These nerve fibers ache with each pulse of blood flowing through the blood vessels, resulting in the throbbing pain associated with migraine headache.

In patients with asthma, irritated nerves controlling the air passages fire off signals that constrict the muscles of the airway and swell the airway lining. Airflow to the lungs decreases, and patients wheeze. In patients with nasal stuffiness, irritated and damaged nerves swell the lining of the nasal passages, blocking the nose.

We could continue to examine the role of nerve damage in numerous other allergic illnesses, but I think the examples I discussed show how all these diverse illnesses can share the same cause—nerve irritation and damage caused by neuroexcitatory and neurotoxic food chemicals.

Different Strokes for Different Folks

Different patients exhibit different symptoms when they eat or drink the chemicals we ask them to avoid. Some experience diarrhea, some have headaches, some get hives, while still others suffer from wheezing or stuffy noses. Why do allergic people show such variation in symptoms? I believe that genetics and injury account for the difference.

In my practice, I treat many families with several allergy-prone members, and I am amazed by the similarity in symptoms within each family. In some, painful migraine headaches are common to many members. In other families, headaches are as rare as a Minnesota summer without mosquitoes, but eczema affects both parents and children. Some gene or combination of genes dictates a weakness for headaches or eczema. In other words, I think these patients have a genetic predisposition for certain illnesses.

I am convinced that injury is another major reason why patients' symptoms appear where they do. Many of our food-sensitive patients experience severe headache pain that begins in an area of the neck that has been injured by whiplash. Those with arthritis experience painful aching in their arthritic joints when they ignore their diet. Patients with intestinal inflammatory diseases such as chronic ulcerative colitis or Crohn's disease find that dietary chemicals stimulate their abdominal distress. The thought that allergy works through the nerves weakened by genetics or injury helps to explain why all these symptoms occur.

Allergy does not cause whiplash, arthritis, and inflammatory bowel disease, but it aggravates them. Allergy is a despicable bully because it is attracted to areas of injury, where it intensifies the pain and discomfort that already exist. That explains why many patients with illnesses that are not caused by allergy are so frequently helped by allergy treatment. Treating allergy chases away the bully.

We have examined the role of acid foods, MSG, and the aspartic acid of low-calorie sweeteners in causing patients' illnesses. One further chemical must be included in this group, and we will meet it in the next section: refined sugar.

Refined Sugar

As I recall, I was feeling content. I had my diet in place. It was complicated, but it worked well. It was true that at first, my patients rebelled against the elimination of favorite foods, but later they praised the diet's effectiveness. I knew I needed to learn more about the components of the diet—MSG, acidic foods, and aspartic acid—but that was gradually happening. All in all, I was satisfied.

But there were sour notes in my symphony of content. One sour note involved my colleagues. Word that I was actively treating patients for food allergy with a new diet was gradually spreading among them, and some were not impressed. To many of my fellow allergists, patients who complain of food allergies and doctors who claim they can treat them are about as welcome as a mass murderer at a convention of homicide detectives.

After all, allergists think that food allergy is mysterious and almost impossible to diagnose and treat. I claimed otherwise: it could be diagnosed and treated if allergists paid attention to certain dietary chemicals. In addition, many allergists believe that most complaints of food allergy spring from the mistaken thoughts of mentally unstable patients with overstimulated imaginations. I claimed that was untrue. I said that my patients were right in believing they suffered from allergies to foods.

Current teaching insists that food allergy is rare and can be diagnosed only by elaborate feeding and avoidance trials. I teach that food allergy frequently plagues patients and that it can be diagnosed using patient histories and skin tests.

I can't say I was ostracized by my fellow allergists, but I certainly was not riding high in their respect and admiration. As much as the next person, I want to be liked by my colleagues, and their reaction to my teachings hurt me. The ultimate blow to my ego came when my nurses attended a lecture for nursing staff from many of the local allergy offices. The speaker poked fun at doctors who treated food allergy by describing a local allergist who had devised a "crazy diet for his mentally unstable patients." Although the speaker didn't mention me by name, it was obvious who he was talking about.

My nurses were shocked. When they told me about the incident, it became clear that my colleagues regarded my work in food allergy as falling somewhere between incompetence and quackery.

In addition, the food allergy symphony struck another discordant note. While avoiding MSG, acidic foods, and aspartic acid helped my patients avoid many headaches, diarrhea episodes, skin rashes, and many other allergic illnesses, it wasn't preventing them all. Some patients still experienced plenty of discomfort.

In the back of my mind I knew there must be other offending foods, but the front of my mind wasn't interested. It didn't want to deal with any more additions to the diet. The back of my mind eventually won out, and another dietary chemical made its way onto the list of things to be eliminated—but only after being forcibly brought to my attention by the same friend who forced me to recognize the harmful effects of MSG.

Can Refined Sugar Be Troublesome?

John and I often sat at his kitchen table settling the affairs of the world and sharing personal experiences. We often talked about John's dreadful cluster headaches as we shared thoughts. I wanted desperately to help free him from the pain of these headaches I described earlier, a searing pain he could not stop but could relieve only by inhaling pure oxygen.

I mentioned our attempts to treat John with allergy shots; in addition, he avoided acidic foods, low-calorie sweeteners, and MSG. John was sure these dietary chemicals precipitated his dreadful cluster headaches, but he still suffered a lot of them. We were missing some other factor that also had to be causing them. What this "other factor" was eluded us—until John found it.

One night as we were sitting at the table, John said, "Bill, I think I've spotted something that causes my headaches."

"Great, John. What is it?" I asked.

"Sugar."

"Oh, come on, John," I retorted in disbelief. "Lots of really elegant studies have looked at sugar and found it doesn't cause any of the illnesses popular folklore blames it for. It's been accused of making kids hyperactive and irritable, and that theory's been shot down often enough. You've got to be wrong."

"I don't think so, Bill. I love sugar. I could eat half a pound of candy at a sitting if someone left a bowlful nearby," he confessed. "I've been wondering if the sugar might have some bearing on my headaches, so I did a little experimenting. I found that if I eat more than two sugar cookies a day, I wake up with a cluster headache. But one or two cookies—no headache."

"John, that's hard to believe," I said, shaking my head. "You've tried this experiment more than once?"

"Yes," he assured me. "Cluster headaches each time."

Now, for me, an auto accident, the end of the world, and the idea of adding another chemical to the diet were equally attractive. I dreaded telling my patients that, in addition to giving up foods high in citric acids, MSG, and low-calorie sweeteners, they'd have to avoid sweets. I could guess how they would react to that charming news. I also dreaded to think what my fellow allergists would say about my putting stock in the sugar-is-bad folklore. Why me?

Then I began to remember that other patients had told me they thought their headaches, diarrhea, and hives might be due to sugar. Each time, I'd dismissed their observations and even argued against them; now I decided I needed to at least consider the possibility.

For the next several weeks I listened closely to my patients for signs that sugar caused their illnesses, and surprisingly the signs were there. When I asked those patients who were using the diet but were still experiencing hives, headaches, and abdominal cramps to avoid sugar, many improved remarkably. Even more amazing, their symptoms recurred when they returned to using sugar. Another chemical joined our diet!

Refined Sugar in the Diet

Refined sugar does not hide in the diet; it announces its presence like a garishly painted clown. We find it everywhere. Unless sweetened by one of the low-calorie sweeteners, any deliciously sweet manufactured food or beverage contains sugar. A partial list of these foods and beverages includes cakes, pies, candies, sweet rolls, fudge, breakfast cereal, carbonated and noncarbonated beverages, jellies, jams, ketchup, salad dressings, ice cream, sweetened yogurt, and sweetened juices. You will have no trouble adding to this list.

You can determine which foods contain large amounts of refined sugar by reading the list of ingredients on processed foods and beverages. Laws require food processors to list certain ingredients on the label, including sugar, with the ingredient making up the highest percentage listed first and the others listed in decreasing order. You will be surprised at the number of foods and beverages that list sugar as one of the first few ingredients.

Recognizing sugar on the list of ingredients can sometimes be difficult, since it comes in many forms and travels under many different aliases. The following is a list of common ones:

Granulated sugar (refined white sugar in granulated form)

Powdered sugar (refined white sugar in powdered form)

Turbinado sugar (partially refined sugar)

Brown sugar (sugar containing molasses-flavored syrup)

Invert sugar (sugar processed with hot acid or enzymes)

Levulose or fructose (made from invert sugar)

Dextrose or corn sugar (made from invert sugar)

Lactose (milk sugar)

Maltose (sugar made from starch using yeast)

Corn syrup (partially refined starch from corn)

Molasses (partially refined sugar from plants)

Honey (refined plant sugar collected by bees)

Maple sugar and syrup (sugar from maple tree sap)

Symptoms of Sugar Intolerance

Excess sugar affects my patients in much the same way that an excess of MSG, aspartic acid, or acidic foods does. All can cause similar symptoms, including hives, wheezing, diarrhea, headaches, or another of the host of illnesses that afflict food-sensitive patients. In addition, like a gang of thieves where each member specializes in performing a particular crime, each of these chemicals seems to predominate in causing a particular symptom or set of symptoms.

I am extremely familiar with MSG's ability in sensitive patients to precipitate bloating and brutal headaches. Sugar also causes both symptoms—remember the cluster headaches John endured. I am also impressed by the ability of citric acid and its fellow acids to provoke the itching of hives and eczema. Sugar also participates in causing these symptoms. Sugar's prime effect seems to be a particularly strong impact on the nerve center of the body—the brain.

Hyperactivity and Sugar

Hyperactivity is a distressingly common and disabling affliction. In our modern world, where education is so highly prized, hyperactivity is a dreadful curse that impedes the ability to learn. The hyperactive child cannot sit still long enough to be taught, cannot remain quiet long enough to study. Saddest of all, he or she cannot sit still long enough for a loving parent to cuddle. Hyperactivity is a crippling handicap.

Although most of us are aware that hyperactivity affects many children, few realize that some adults are similarly victimized. Like children, they find it hard to remain calm long enough to complete complex tasks or to enjoy meaningful human interactions.

My patients tell me about numerous instances of food-induced hyperactivity. A good illustration is Mary's family of two lively little girls. By the time I walked into the examining room for our first consultation, they had partially demolished it. Tammie was on top of the examining table, tearing the paper to shreds, and Tracie was trying to haul the footstool out the door in spite of Mary's desperate attempts to keep her from doing so.

Because I see hyperactivity so frequently in my little patients, I quickly spotted it in the girls. A sure sign was Tracie scampering around the room like a squirrel in a cage. A second sign—the look on Mary's face that told me she was sorry for the disturbance but was powerless to stop it—reinforced my thought.

Mary is powerless. You can spank a child you love only so many times before you cannot force yourself to do it again—especially when deep down you feel the child cannot help his or her behavior. I am one of those who believe the fault does not lie with the child (nor does it lie with the parent). It often lies in the diet.

Mary's primary-care doctor sent the girls to see me because of their eczema. After testing them, and after we discussed the eczema, I also raised the subject of their hyperactivity. Mary seemed hesitant to discuss it. Like many parents of hyperactive children, I believe she had given up hope that she could do anything to stop it.

We discussed dietary changes, and I stressed reduction of both acidic foods, to help the eczema, and refined sugar, to see if it would have an affect on the hyperactivity. When Mary and the girls returned in three months to review their progress, she was far more willing to talk. And my office wasn't demolished.

"How did the girls like the diet, Mary?"

"Not at all, Dr. Walsh. In fact, they hate it," she admitted.

"That's not strange, Mary. Lots of our patients complain about having to avoid the foods they love. Does it help the girls?" I asked.

"It's very helpful. As long as we stick to it, their skin is almost clear."

Then she told me that the only time they had broken away from the diet was at a birthday party at school. Sodas, cake, and ice cream were served, and both little girls stuffed themselves.

"Next day both were full of hives and broke out in eczema," she reported. "I was surprised at the lesson it taught them, though. Neither of them will eat sugary foods now."

I wasn't surprised. Even two- and three-year-old children will avoid sweet-tasting treats if they connect them with discomfort and pain. That's why I instruct parents not to force children to follow our diet. If the diet works and the parents point out the link between food and discomfort, children will usually avoid the offending foods.

In fact, I am often astonished by the children who intuitively avoid eating or drinking foods high in illness-producing chemicals, a habit they start long before I first see them. If "Johnny, drink your juice" provokes a mother-child battle, there's a good possibility that Johnny recognizes that he and juice mix poorly.

"What about sugar, Mary?" I asked.

"That part really surprised me, Dr. Walsh. Tammie and Tracie are both much calmer on the diet. Even my mother-in-law notices, and the girls' teacher is delighted."

She told me that after the birthday party, the girls' behavior deteriorated. For the next two days they were unmanageable, jumping from one thing to another without stopping, and driving their teacher wild.

They showed this same behavior when Mary's father-in-law brought candy to the house. "They got into it when we weren't watching," she said. "Now we keep no more sweets at home, and their teacher watches to see they do not eat sweets in the classroom."

The only exception I make to the "let the children manage their own diet" rule is hyperactivity. Children often do not recognize that they are hyperactive, so they fail to see the link between their behavior and the diet. Parents must be able to recognize this cause-and-effect relationship and stress avoiding the foods that cause it, or children will not follow the diet.

"Did you try the diet yourself, Mary?" I asked.

"Yes, I did," she said. "As a child I was hyperactive, and now I often have days when I'm tired and irritable and can't seem to think straight. [My patients refer to this as being "spacey" or "spaced out."] Now I know I'll have days like that if I eat too much sugar. I wish someone had told me about sugar and hyperactivity when I was young."

I do, too. I feel sorry for the many children—and adults—who never have a chance at scholastic achievement or many of life's other rewards because of their hyperactivity. Even love and cuddling are almost impossible for children who cannot sit still long enough to be held. I firmly believe that their unmanageable behavior springs not from an innate and hateful defiance, but from the hyperstimulation of the various food chemicals—especially sugar.

Mary told me she was delighted with the diet's effect on her own symptoms, but she admitted she found it hard to give up sugar. A genuine craving for sugar often overcomes her. In fact, when she took it out of her diet, she suffered miserable symptoms for five days. "I felt tired and irritable, I couldn't sleep, my hands shook, and I had a horrible headache."

Sugar Craving

Many other patients share Mary's experience when she eliminated sugar from her diet—nearly intolerable symptoms of withdrawal. About one out of four or five of my patients craves sugar; they suffer dreadfully when they eliminate it. Their symptoms vary and may include shaky hands, muscle aches and pains, perspiration, sleeplessness, and striking irritability; in other words, they feel terrible.

These withdrawal symptoms form a substantial barrier to treating patients who crave sugar. It is hard for them to recognize that sugar avoidance, which brings such pain, is necessary to control their headaches, body aches and pains, diarrhea, and other distresses.

It does, though. Many of my patients find that excess sugar makes their noses stuff and their heads hurt; hardly a day goes by when patients fail to mention the ill effects of too many treats.

When patients crave sugar so much that elimination makes them suffer unpleasant withdrawal symptoms, denial often comes into play. They often deny even the possibility that sugar could be causing symptoms. My staff and I have found that this craving and denial are signposts pointing to the foods that are almost certainly a major cause of our patients' problems. We try to identify food cravings so we can teach our patients to be cautious of these foods or food chemicals.

I mention food craving because we encounter it so frequently and find it so difficult to counter. In many cases patients fight our diagnosis for years and continue to suffer until they accept it. It typically takes three years for especially resistant patients to come around.

A good example is Judy, a thirty-five-year-old emergency room nurse I have been treating for migraines for several years. At the outset she tried to eliminate refined sugar, suffered overwhelming withdrawal headaches and irritability, and decided sugar was not to blame. After three years, on one of her regular follow-up visits, I asked: "How are you doing, Judy?"

"Really well, Dr. Walsh. My migraines are fine as long as I get my shots every two weeks." (We will discuss how allergy injections can help relieve food symptoms later in this book.)

"What about your diet? I asked. "Do any foods bring on the headaches?"

"I have to avoid tomatoes, oranges, and MSG entirely or I get bad headaches," she said. "I also have to watch potatoes and cheese, and I can only have pizza if I don't eat any bad food for two days before the pizza."

When I asked, "What about sugar?" I was surprised at Judy's answer.

"I've eliminated it from my diet altogether. Once I start to eat sugar, I can't stop and I end up irritable, I can't think clearly, and I get hit with a horrible headache."

You do not make friends when you say "I told you so," so I didn't. But I remembered three years back when Judy said the diet was stupid and sugar didn't bother her. Eventually she became aware that sugar was the culprit, but she suffered a long time before recognizing it. Perhaps her story will help others with sugar craving realize something they don't want to face.

I often reflect on my experiences with sugar. I was reluctant to add it to the elimination diet—another chemical that many of my patients must avoid. However, together my patients and I learned that it must be eliminated to truly control their distressing symptoms.

Sugar's effects on the brain—sugar craving, hyperactivity, "spacey thinking"—also forced me to confront the effect of all allergies, especially the food chemical allergies, on the central nervous system. I believe that brain effects are potent. This allergy/brain connection ensures sugar and its related food chemicals a permanent place in the elimination diet.

We reviewed the four food chemicals that my patients must avoid or limit in their diets. Now is the time to review certain foods and beverages whose place is less certain but perhaps very important in an elimination diet for allergic patients.

Foods, Beverages, and Supplements

In our discussion of foods and beverages that cause patient reactions, I touched only lightly on several that we should now consider further. We eat these food and beverages frequently; when consuming them, sensitive patients must exercise caution.

Corn

Corn deserves special attention because we eat it so frequently and also because it causes major allergy symptoms. For many of my patients it provokes the same symptoms as the food chemicals we discussed—refined sugar, acid foods, MSG, and low-calorie sweeteners.

Many patients are allergic to corn and show this allergy by a positive skin test to corn. However, in other patients who react to corn, the cause is a mystery. When we skin-test these patients for corn, their test is negative. This negative test indicates that the protein in corn is not to blame (allergy to protein is the usual cause of a positive skin test), but that the reaction spouted from a different seed.

Perhaps we can find where this seed was planted by following its history. From this history we learn that today's corn plant was developed from an American weed used thousands of years ago for food. Our forefathers planted successive generations of corn, and as they selected the seed they would use for the next planting, their choices made corn slowly but surely change. For instance, the ear that was originally the size of a strawberry grew to the modern seed-bearing hulk we buy at the grocery store.

Features other than size also changed. As each generation of farmers selected corn that gave larger size, they must also have selected corn with improved flavor. Where does some of this flavor originate? From MSG.

We know that MSG gives both natural and processed foods a robust and pleasant taste, and corn is naturally rich in this free amino acid. The pleasant taste sought by our ancestors meant they kept selecting and propagating corn with higher MSG content. This high content may account for the unpleasant reactions some of my patients suffer.

What sensitive patients should avoid. I find the ramifications of corn allergy disturbing. Corn, the world's most widely distributed food crop, is found in countless products, including breakfast cereals, cornmeal, corn bread, corn starch, corn syrup, crackers, popcorn, tortillas, and numerous others. Obviously, eliminating corn from the diet poses a terrible hardship. A frequent question my patients ask is whether they must avoid all corn products.

While I can't be entirely sure, I don't think so. MSG-sensitive people are primarily concerned with corn's MSG content. I suspect that MSG may be lost during some forms of corn processing to make chips, syrup, and other products. Therefore, unless MSG is added after baking, cereals, crackers, breads, and similar products are probably acceptable for patients sensitive to MSG. Isn't it a shame that we cannot determine the MSG content of a corn-derived food from the foods list of ingredients?

Thorough boiling may flush MSG out of corn that we prepare at home. This may be the reason why so many allergy patients find that corn on the cob causes them grief. If corn is cut from the cob and then boiled, or boiled on the cob until soft, allergy patients often seem able to tolerate it. With this preparation method, each of the corn seeds is cut open, allowing the MSG in the seed to be dissolved and dissipated into the boiling water.

The anticipation with which we await the late summer harvest of delicious sweet corn—and the widespread popularity of this grain product—combine to hide its effects on allergy patients, who often fail to notice their corn allergy until they are warned to watch for symptoms after they eat it.

I share my patients' love of corn on the cob and their distress after eating it. In fact, the bloating and abdominal pains I suffer after a delicious meal of corn on the cob first brought this food allergy to my attention.

Unfortunately, the potential for corn on the cob to cause suffering is shared by popcorn. Again, this is a food that has not been boiled to reduce its MSG content.

Besides baking and boiling, MSG in corn and other vegetables also can be reduced by storing the food for at least twenty-four hours before preparation; stored foods contain less MSG than fresh foods. I suspect that the free MSG is converted into proteins as it sits in the refrigerator.

Peanuts

I know that many patients would more readily accept the need to avoid popcorn if they could substitute a crunchy handful of peanuts as they watch a ball game or snack at a party. Unfortunately, for many patients this substitution brings regrettable symptoms.

My staff and I learned about the potential for peanuts to cause harm from patients who gave up popcorn when they found it made them feel sick. Many of them told us that when they replaced popcorn with peanuts, they experienced the same discomfort. I know that I suffer uncomfortable symptoms from both foods if I eat more than I can tolerate.

It is surprising that pain and discomfort can be caused by such an important food source. Like corn, peanuts are a major food crop; seventeen million metric tons are grown per year and processed as peanut butter or simply roasted and sold at sporting events, circuses, etc., and as at-home snacks.

Also like corn, the peanut has long been used as a human food. It is known to have existed as early as 950 B.C. in South America, and early explorers in the sixteenth century found its use widespread throughout Mexico and South America.

The peanut may be similar to corn in another way. Although I was unable to determine the exact MSG content of the peanut from my reference materials, I suspect that as a member of the pea family (hence the name peanut) it contains significant amounts of MSG. In fact, peas contain more MSG than corn. Most of my patients tolerate boiled peas—the boiling process must reduce the level of MSG. Unfortunately, the processing of shelled and unshelled peanuts does not seem to confer similar benefits.

Oddly enough, many of my patients who cannot eat a handful of peanuts do seem to tolerate peanut butter. Perhaps some step in the processing of peanuts into peanut butter inactivates or removes MSG. On the other hand, they may eat fewer peanuts when it is in the form of peanut butter and so do not exceed their tolerance for peanuts. We tell our patients to try eating peanut butter; they can continue to eat it as long as it does not stimulate symptoms.

A word of caution: People who experience life-threatening symptoms (e.g., breathing difficulty, hives, loss of consciousness, or other severe reactions) from eating peanuts should never try to eat this food in any form.

Beans also can cause distressing symptoms in the allergic person, and I have personal experience with some beans. Every once in a while I have a meal with green beans or other bean products that have not been thoroughly boiled. They have a somewhat crunchy texture, and this clue to their less than completely cooked nature saves me much pain if I heed it. If I eat them anyway, I experience an MSG-type reaction (my bad knee swells, my stomach burns, and I sleep poorly at night). A good, hard boiling until the beans are soft—even mushy—spares me all this trouble. It also may spare you.

Alcoholic Beverages

My patients often ask me about drinking alcoholic beverages. Unfortunately, because distillers and wine producers are not required to provide any information on liquor labels other than alcohol content, I must base my advice about alcoholic beverages on meager data and much guessing. However, certain facts serve as a partial guide.

As mentioned earlier, because fermentation of any food or beverage releases MSG as the food protein breaks down, you can expect to find MSG in any alcoholic beverage. My primary advice is to drink in moderation so that you do not accumulate an excess of MSG.

Some alcoholic beverages seem worse than others. Corn-based liquors such as bourbon cause many of my patients great distress; they seem to tolerate grain-based beverages such as scotch much better. The same is true for beer. American beer is often brewed from corn and seems to be poorly tolerated by my patients compared to barley-based beers such as many German and American ales and lagers.

I caution my patients to avoid using any mixer other than water; some mixes contain high amounts of sugar and acid.

I also tell my patients to be extremely careful of brandy and wines, especially the red wines. Because brandy and wine are fermented products and fermentation releases MSG, and because both contain the citric and tartaric acid of grapes, their combination of acid/MSG is particularly bothersome to many of my patients.

Yogurt

Yogurt is produced from milk by fermenting it with bacteria. Unfortunately, this fermentation releases some of the glutamic and aspartic acids that help make up the milk's protein, and both of these amino acids irritate my patients. The amount of these free amino acids probably varies depending on the fermentation process, as is the case with cheese—the more fermented (aged) the cheese, the more elevated the MSG content. The more fermented the yogurt, the more MSG it contains. Lacking information on the free amino acid content of various yogurt brands, I cannot tell you which brand may be lowest in these acids and thus best for patients with allergy.

I suspect that the levels of free aspartic acid and MSG in yogurt are lower than in aged cheese. Most of my patients can tolerate a limited amount in their diet; however, eating a lot of it could be a great mistake. It also would be inadvisable to eat flavored yogurts, especially those that contain aspartame or citrus; the effect of the sugar and acid content combined with MSG and aspartic acid could lead to uncomfortable symptoms.

The Cabbage Family

The number of my patients who are sensitive to cabbage, cauliflower, broccoli, and Brussels sprouts surprises me. My nursing staff and I took an informal survey and found that many of our patients suffer symptoms from either corn or the cabbage family. Interestingly enough, most patients reacted to one or the other but not to both. I caution you that this was an unscientific survey, and I have no idea why this was the result. Nor do I know why so many of my patients react to the cabbage family. Watch for this allergy. Boiling these foods well may allow you to eat them, even if you react to them when you eat them uncooked (such as in coleslaw).

Caffeinated Beverages

Patients often ask me whether caffeinated beverages such as coffee can give rise to some of the symptoms they experience. I am hesitant to say yes or no, mostly because I don't know.

Skin tests help me diagnose the cause of allergic disorders; they point to these causes like signposts point out the correct road to a city. Unfortunately, because there is no skin test for caffeine, there is no signpost telling me if caffeine is a problem for my patients.

A traveler on a road with no signposts must rely on a best guess as to which direction to take. Similarly, I must rely on guesswork to answer this question. However, sometimes an event occurs that leaves such a strong impression that it influences the direction this guesswork takes. Such an event happened while I was visiting a dear friend in the hospital where he was recovering from hip replacement surgery. Al and I attended medical school together, and we now practice in the same town. In the course of our conversation, he asked me if any of my patients had reported unusual symptoms associated with coffee. After confessing that I was unsure of the role of coffee in causing allergic symptoms, I asked him what prompted the question, and our conversation went something like this.

"Well, Bill, a weird thing happened to me recently," he began, with a satisfied look on his face.

"Tell me about it, Al," I said, curious to find out what he might have to tell me about coffee.

"Peculiar things have been happening with my vision lately," he said. "Spots float in and out, flashes of light come and go, and sometimes part of my vision is hazy and I can't see very well. I keep thinking I've got something in my eye and try to brush it away. It's really upsetting and probably dangerous, especially when I'm driving at night."

My recounting of this experience indicates the tendency for caffeine—in coffee—to cause symptoms. Al suspected that coffee caused his symptoms, which were those of the aura (vision disturbance) that often precedes a migraine headache, and confirmed this suspicion when he stopped drinking coffee and his symptoms disappeared. Luckily for Al, the headache did not follow the aura, as it does in so many unfortunate people who suffer migraine's throbbing pain. But he was perceptive enough to realize that his symptoms probably represented a migraine aura and to remove coffee from his diet.

With caffeine elimination, the vision disturbances disappeared. He further confirmed his suspicions during a "curbstone consultation" with a neurologist. The neurologist agreed with his suspicions. (A curbstone consultation occurs when a doctor informally consults with another doctor for personal advice without seeing him in his office. Doctors go to great lengths to treat themselves instead of seeing another doctor.)

As you can imagine, this experience makes me very suspicious of caffeine. Although Al's aura never grew to a rip-roaring headache, I see no reason why it wouldn't in people more susceptible to this cruel pain. My own experiences with caffeine further raise my suspicions. It causes abdominal cramps and burning if I take it. I must avoid caffeine.

My advice is, if you react to foods, be very careful of caffeine. If you do not suffer symptoms from caffeine, enjoy the tasty beverages it flavors.

Food Supplements

Many food supplements are marketed for people on diets or for those who want to improve their strength and endurance for sports and exercise. These supplements worry me. Many are derived from proteins that are hydrolyzed (broken down) into their constituent amino acids. This preparation frees both aspartic and glutamic acids, and we have already discussed the effects of these amino acids. I ask my patients sensitive to these amino acids to avoid such supplements.

Vitamins

The question my patients ask most frequently is: "If I cut out all these foods, where do I get my vitamins?" The answer is obvious when you examine the foods that are acceptable in the diet. The many fresh fruits, vegetables, and meats that are allowed contain all the vitamins you need for proper nutrition. And, conversely, many of the foods we eliminate from the diet contain little or no nutritional value and do not threaten your vitamin needs.

Many people supplement their diet with extra vitamins—in most cases, the one-a-day type. For many of my patients this is unwise; supplemental vitamins often make them ill. I confess to taking vitamins from time to time, but a week of taking vitamins makes me tired and nauseated.

I am not sure why vitamin supplements cause so much discomfort. One vitamin, vitamin C, is usually packaged with citric acid. Pharmacists tell me that vitamin C needs to be combined with citric acid to prevent deterioration and inactivation.

Many of my patients also react poorly to vitamins that do not contain vitamin C. In some cases I believe they react because the vitamins contain yeast as a source of some of the vitamins. It is not difficult to conclude that those who are allergic to yeast would develop pain and discomfort from ingesting it in vitamin supplements.

In examining my own reactions to vitamins and hearing the experiences of my patients who are sensitive to vitamins, I wonder if vitamins cause an MSG-type reaction in sensitive people. The bloating, diarrhea, rashes, abdominal pain, and other symptoms shared by me and others are typical of MSG reactions. This is not surprising, since labels on a number of vitamins specify that they are complexed to glutamic acid (MSG).

Symptoms arising from taking vitamins make me wonder whether we should reexamine their value. They may not be as harmless as we think. It's like the owner of a Volkswagen Beetle who, unsatisfied with its ruggedness and reliability, wants it to accelerate like a dragster. So he drives it to the airport and fills the tank with jet engine fuel. Much to his chagrin, he finds that instead of accelerating better, the car barely operates at all because it was never designed to run on jet fuel.

Maybe vitamins are like jet fuel for the body. Instead of improving its operation, perhaps they pose a threat we do not recognize.

Salt

Strictly speaking, salt is not a food; it is a seasoning. However, no book about food allergy would be complete without mentioning the effect of salt on patients with allergy, because many of them notice that excess salt increases their allergic symptoms.

How does salt cause increased symptoms for my patients? In certain people salt seems to promote fluid accumulation, and this may aggravate the bloating effect of many food reactions—a consequence my patients and I experience when our diets are too heavily loaded with foods and beverages we tolerate poorly.

If excess salt is a source of discomfort for you, it would be wise to limit your intake of salty foods and refrain from adding salt to your food.

In our discussion of food allergy we have paid special attention to food allergy caused by acid foods, MSG, low-calorie sweeteners, and refined sugar. Now is an appropriate time to look closely at the symptoms food allergy causes, again stressing those symptoms caused by food chemicals. Of all the food allergies, the ones generated by food chemicals are the most frequent.

Putting Our Information to Use

Patients Who Suffer Food-Chemical Symptoms

To help you understand the symptoms caused by MSG, low-calorie sweeteners, and excess refined sugar and acid, imagine you are accompanying me in my office and visiting with some of the patients I treat. All of the patients I introduce you to suffer symptoms from food chemicals. Through their experiences we can hear firsthand how food allergy, especially food-chemical allergy, affects their lives.

Although I will try to focus primarily on food-chemical allergy, I will not limit our discussion to only this type of food allergy, since patients can be affected by more than one type of food allergy.

Janie Suffers Severe Headaches

"My main problem is headaches, and they are awful. They start in the back of my head and move across the top of my head into my forehead and eyes. They throb painfully, so bad that before my neurologist prescribed Imitrex [an excellent prescription migraine pain reliever], I had to go to bed in a dark room, desperately hoping I could sleep them away. Sometimes that didn't work and the pain lasted for days."

Janie's headaches are relieved with allergy injections, and she helped herself by correcting some bad mite and mold exposures at home. One of her most effective actions involved tearing out a shower wall that was moldy.

She continues, "I have to be very careful of what I eat, especially foods such as cheese. Cheese sets off a severe migraine headache very quickly after I eat it. One of my worst headaches came after an Italian dinner that featured lots of cheese. Tomatoes and sauces with tomato also cause headaches, but these headaches develop hours after I eat."

We can learn much from Janie's story. Cheese, which contains MSG, brings Jane a rapidly appearing reaction, resulting in a severely painful migraine headache. Tomato brings on a delayed food symptom, headache, probably an allergy to the protein of tomato assisted by the tomato's naturally elevated levels of acid and MSG.

Joy Experiences Mouth Sores

Joy's story shows that foods can cause multiple symptoms.

She begins, "My worst troubles come from oranges. Whenever I eat them or drink orange juice, my nose runs and my mouth breaks out in sores. These sores take days to heal, sometimes several weeks. Other acidic foods, such as grapefruit and berries, do not cause as much trouble as long as I do not eat or drink too much of them.

"One more thing bothers me: I love the taste of beer, but whenever I drink it, I bloat up."

Not only do many of my patients bloat from foods or beverages, I also bloat from foods, especially those containing MSG. If I eat these foods, I develop a great thirst and drink a lot of water, which pools in my tissues. The next day, like the comic-strip cat Garfield, my scale scolds me for gaining five to ten pounds. It takes three days before I lose the extra weight.

Many people claim that acidic foods cause mouth ulcers and canker sores of the lips. As I have already mentioned, my experiences and those of my patients convince me that these observations are correct: acidic foods and drinks either cause or aggravate mouth sores. As Joy mentioned, among the acidic foods, oranges seem unusually potent in causing these sores and ulcers.

Many of my patients tell me about bloating after drinking beer. As I suffer the same symptom from certain beers, I understand their frustrations at being denied this beverage. As a doctor, it helps me to share the symptoms that plague my patients; sympathizing is no effort.

Rachel Feels Ill

Rachel's story is instructive. She lived with headaches for years before I treated her. Like many of my patients, she suffers from two different types of headaches. One, which involves sinus pain, penetrates deeply into her forehead and quickly jumps to the back of her head. A second migrainelike headache throbs painfully behind her right eye.

Because her pain involves the back of her head and radiates into her neck muscles, her previous doctors had told her that she suffered from tension headaches. I know that tension causes or aggravates headaches, but even tense people can suffer headaches caused by allergy. Too many of my patients have been treated for tension without the medical care-giver considering that allergy might be playing a contributing role. I wish they thought of allergy as often as they think about tension as a probable headache cause and not overlook allergy so readily.

Rachel comments, "My worst food allergy concerns MSG and diet sodas. Both give me a migraine headache within minutes, and the headache is dreadful. I also feel very nauseated and ill."

"Do any other foods cause you trouble?" I ask.

"Yes, potato- and tomato-based foods make me feel sick, my nose stuffy, and my stomach ache, but only if I eat too many of them. If I eat these foods only two to three days a week I'm okay, but if I eat them several days in a row, I'm stuffy and my stomach hurts."

Rachel adds, "I often get the same sickness, stomach pain, and headache when I eat at a restaurant. I'm not sure why that happens."

"I suspect the cook flavored your food with MSG, Rachel," I reply. "When you eat out, remember to select a simple meal such as a steak or fish with no sauce or breading and ask the cook to put no seasoning of any type on it. Often restaurant staff members are unaware that the seasoning they use contains MSG, so telling them not to use MSG doesn't always help. Tell your server to 'just cook it and bring it.' That's the best way to avoid MSG flavoring in your meal."

Rachel reacts quickly to MSG and low-calorie sweeteners, and small amounts are able to provoke these sudden symptoms. The acids in tomatoes and potatoes also make her sick, but these are delayed symptoms, and she must eat a larger quantity of these foods to bring on her headaches, stomach aches, and sickness.

Jim Also Suffers Headaches

Our next patient shares Rachel's sensitivity to MSG and low-calorie sweeteners. Jim came to the office to restart allergy injections to dust, mold, and pollen; an insurance policy change forced him to stop this treatment. Without these injections, however, his daily headaches returned, with all the pain and discomfort he suffered when I first saw him. Now, with a new insurance policy in place, he can return for treatment.

"MSG and low-calorie sweeteners make my head hurt," Jim says. Most of the time I feel the pain behind my eyes, and it throbs painfully. MSG headaches come on quickly after I eat something with MSG, but the headaches that follow diet soda usually come on hours later. I can't drink sodas with sugar either because I get the same headaches.

"I tried substituting fruit juices for the sodas, but my stomach burns and the burning travels right up to my throat. It seems I can drink only water and milk."

Jim advises the reader, "I've learned to watch out for what I eat, and I think you should do the same if you have headaches or stomach trouble. But do not think only of your diet when you look for the things that make you sick. The air that you breathe at work and at home can be equally important or more important."

Megan Suffers Diarrhea

Megan suffers diarrhea if she does not carefully restrict her diet. This diarrhea embarrasses her; I will let her tell you why.

"I have a severe sensitivity to MSG that causes an explosive diarrhea. If I am eating out in a restaurant with friends and I eat any by mistake, I have to run right away to the bathroom and stay there until it's over, sometimes for an hour. My friends are forced to wait for me. I feel so embarrassed.

"Tomatoes, onions, cucumbers, and cabbage also cause diarrhea, although only if I eat more than I tolerate. When I eat any of these foods, I eat only small amounts."

What We Learned from These Patients

Janie, Joy, Rachel, Jim, and Megan taught us the following lessons:

1. *Food allergy often does not exist in isolation.* These patients showed us that food allergy often does not exist in isolation but in combination with significant allergy to dust mites, mold, pollen, and pets. Although in our visits we concentrated on food-chemical allergy, we treat each of these patients with allergy injections for environmental allergy. To give them relief from their suffering, we must blend treatment for diet and environmental allergies.

2. *People often suffer from allergy to both the particular food and to the chemicals it contains.* Their stories also teach us that people often suffer symptoms from foods and food chemicals, both right away and hours later. For instance, Megan suffers immediate diarrhea when she eats MSG but delayed diarrhea to tomatoes, onions, cucumbers, and the cabbage family. We commonly find patients sensitive to this combination of allergies to foods and food chemicals.

3. *Food-chemical allergy affects a large number of our patients.* Allergy to acidic foods, refined sugar, low-calorie sweeteners, and MSG affects a large number of our patients to a greater or lesser degree. You

must understand this type of food allergy if you want to understand and treat your own food allergy.

Are these patients right? Are they correctly interpreting their experiences? Can MSG really cause headaches and explosive diarrhea, and make you feel sick?

I believe it can. The best way to let you see the universe of symptoms caused by MSG is to review a study we performed in our office. In the next section, I'll show you what we found.

Symptoms Caused by MSG

Can MSG really cause all the symptoms my patients have mentioned? If it causes these symptoms, are there other symptoms it can cause?

How many symptoms does MSG cause? So often I am surprised by its presence in an allergic symptom. In many cases I would not have suspected MSG if my patients had not told me it caused their symptoms.

In the 1992 report of the Federation of American Societies for Experimental Biology, "Illnesses Caused by MSG," the committee recognized a variety of symptoms caused by MSG, ranging from numbness, burning, and tingling to headache, drowsiness, and weakness.

Could these symptoms affect my own patients? I decided to find out. I designed a study to look at MSG symptoms more closely, and what I found helped me to better anticipate these symptoms and may also help resolve your questions.

I centered my study on the people who best know MSG, my patients. By learning about their experiences, I learned about the unfortunate consequences that arise in sensitive people eating foods prepared with this delicious flavoring agent.

A Study of MSG Symptoms

To learn how MSG affected our patients I used a symptoms check-off list prepared by the MSG Sensitivity Institute, Inc., in Concord, New Hampshire.

My nurses and I asked our patients if they suffered any symptoms from foods flavored with MSG. If they answered yes, we asked them to study the list of symptoms and, to the best of their ability, check off those they experienced. In all, 153 patients told us they reacted to MSG and filled out the form.

The following information summarizes their replies. It lists their symptoms in decreasing order of frequency in each of the symptom categories on the list. As most patients suffered more than one symptom, the number of symptoms adds up to more than the 153 patients questioned.

As you will see, the results of our study of MSG symptoms show their impressive variety and potential for mischief. No area of the body seems immune from its afflictions.

You should keep several cautions in mind as you examine the results of our study. We did not explain each of the symptoms to our patients; we simply asked them to fill out the information to the best of their ability.

If we had questioned each patient individually, I believe the number of reported symptoms would have been much higher—I think we could have brought out symptoms they were overlooking. I believe this would have substantially raised the number of reported symptoms, especially those affecting emotions, mood, and thinking such as depression, anxiety, and disorientation. My patients seem hesitant to admit these symptoms and often will do so only if questioned in a sympathetic manner.

A further caution: we did not feed MSG to these patients, so we did not verify their answers experimentally. However, since the results we obtained are consistent with symptoms described to me by my other MSG-sensitive patients, I do not doubt the following results that we obtained.

NEUROLOGICAL (BRAIN AND PERIPHERAL NERVES)

Type of Symptom	Number Who Reacted (153 patients)
Migraine headache	72
Pressure behind eyes (sinus headache]	56
Lightheadedness	45
Drowsiness	34
Lethargy	20
Dizziness	17
Anxiety	15

Type of Symptom	*Number Who Reacted* *(153 patients)*
Depression	13
Insomnia	12
Disorientation	12
Loss of balance	11
Headache (other than above)	11
Numbness	8
Mental confusion	8
Hyperactivity	8
Panic attacks	7
Slurred speech	5
Behavioral problems in children	3

RESPIRATORY (NOSE, THROAT, AIRWAYS, AND LUNGS)

Type of Symptom	*Number Who Reacted* *(153 patients)*
Runny nose, postnasal drip	67
Sneezing	38
Shortness of breath	33
Asthma	17
Tightness of muscles	16
Chest pain	10

GASTROINTESTINAL (STOMACH, INTESTINES)

Type of Symptom	*Number Who Reacted* *(153 patients)*
Abdominal discomfort or cramping	66
Diarrhea	53
Bloating	49
Irritable bowel	36
Nausea	28
Loss of bowel or bladder control	11
Vomiting	8

SKIN

Type of Symptom	Number Who Reacted (153 patients)
Flushing of face or body	37
Rash	17
Hives	13
Tingling	12
Mouth lesions	7
Extreme dryness of mouth or thirst	3

CARDIAC

Type of Symptom	Number Who Reacted (153 patients)
Tachycardia (rapid heartbeat)	17
Extreme drop in blood pressure	7
Angina	5
Arrhythmia	2

MUSCULAR

Type of Symptom	Number Who Reacted (153 patients)
Flulike achiness	26
Joint pain	15
Stiffness	12
Shaking of body parts	10

VISUAL

Type of Symptom	Number Who Reacted (153 patients)
Difficulty focusing	12
Blurred vision	9

CIRCULATORY

Type of Symptom	*Number Who Reacted (153 patients)*
Swelling	37

Interpretation of Results

Our MSG-sensitive patients gave us illuminating answers. They told us that MSG symptoms can affect any area of the body. Brain and peripheral nerves, stomach and intestines, lungs and air passages, heart and blood vessels, muscles and joints, eyes and skin—all can be affected and frequently are.

If we had asked them about other members of the food chemicals allergy gang—refined sugar, acid foods, and low-calorie sweeteners—I expect that the results would have been similar. Many of our patients tolerate these other food chemicals poorly.

The most important information you can gain from this study concerns the recognition of your own discomfort and pain. If you suffer from one or more of these symptoms, these food chemicals may be the cause or part of the cause.

Take a few minutes and read the results of our study again. It can teach you much about food chemicals allergy.

The obvious answer to MSG sensitivity is to avoid eating MSG. This does not have to be complete avoidance; just avoid eating more than you tolerate. Even the most sensitive patient can tolerate some MSG without suffering.

Although the need to avoid is obvious, actually doing it is difficult. In the next section we will explore some of the problems and pitfalls involved in avoiding MSG.

How to Avoid MSG

You met my patients who suffer symptoms when they use MSG to flavor their food, eat a manufactured food with MSG flavoring purchased from the grocery, or encounter it in a restaurant. You read the results of our questionnaire about MSG symptoms. Now that you know how

MSG-sensitive patients suffer, wouldn't you expect me to give them the following instructions?

"Jim, you are intensely allergic to MSG. This doesn't mean that you must completely avoid it, but you must severely restrict the amount you eat every day. Read every label on the foods you buy, watching for the words 'MSG.' Try to eat no more than one milligram of MSG in any twenty-four hour period."

Or I might say, "Mary, although you are only mildly allergic to MSG, try not to eat more than four milligrams in any twenty-four-hour period. More than four milligrams will most likely set off one of your terrible migraine headaches."

Although you would expect me to give these instructions to every MSG-sensitive patient, I cannot. Two factors stop me:

◇ MSG has more names than Bartholomew Cubbins has hats. If you tried to avoid MSG by checking each food label for MSG or monosodium glutamate, you could still eat a diet high in MSG. Its presence is hidden behind innocent-sounding names that do not contain the words "monosodium glutamate" or the letters "MSG."

◇ Food manufacturers are not required to state on the food label the amount of MSG contained in the food. Without this information, you cannot restrict your dietary intake of MSG to the amount you can tolerate.

Because the amount is not stated, I have been unable to determine how much MSG my severely sensitive patients can tolerate. I also do not know how much MSG my mildly sensitive patients can tolerate. The figures between one and four milligrams that I used above may not even be in the ballpark.

The Names That Hide MSG

In our modern world of consumer rights, you would expect that the foods that contain MSG would be well known and that a sensitive person could identify these foods by reading their labels and eliminating any foods with MSG or monosodium glutamate. I wish this were so.

Unfortunately, even I, who have treated MSG-sensitive patients for years, do not know for sure all the foods that contain this flavoring agent. I also am unsure that I can recognize all the names it hides behind.

In the section "Monosodium Glutamate (Alias MSG)," earlier in this chapter, I provided a 1991 FDA list of foods that contain MSG. The MSG-sensitive patient should also be aware that other lists exist. If you are computer-savvy, you can find these lists by searching the Internet using a search engine and typing in the words "monosodium glutamate." I did this and found the following information from a number of lists; it should assist you in your quest for a diet low in this flavoring. I believe the following information is correct.

Foods That Always Contain MSG

Caseinate
  Calcium caseinate
  Sodium caseinate
Gelatin
Glutamate/glutamic acid
  Monopotassium
    glutamate
  Monosodium
    glutamate

Protein
  Hydrolyzed soy/vegetable/
    etc. protein
  Hydrolyzed protein
  Textured protein
Yeast
  Autolyzed yeast
  Yeast extract
  Yeast food
  Yeast nutrient

Foods That Often Contain MSG
or That Create MSG During Processing

Bouillon
Broth
Carrageenan
Enzymes
  Enzyme-modified foods
Fermented foods and
  beverages

Beer
Bourbon/scotch/whiskey
Brandy/wine
Other alcoholic drinks
Flavors & flavorings
  Natural flavorings
  Natural beef flavoring

Natural chicken flavoring

Natural pork flavoring

Smoke flavoring

Malt

   Barley malt

   Malt extract

   Malt flavoring

Maltodextrin

Pectin

Protease and protease enzymes

Protein

   Protein-fortified foods

   Textured protein

Seasonings

Soy

   Soy extract

   Soy protein

   Soy protein concentrate

   Soy protein isolate

   Soy sauce

Stock

Ultrapasteurized foods

Whey

   Whey protein

   Whey protein concentrate

   Whey protein isolate

Are These Lists Complete?

I am afraid that the answer is probably not. Although the lists may be incomplete, they show you the detective skills you need to safeguard your diet.

A second question also is pertinent. Do all of the food ingredients listed above need to be avoided? Perhaps not. Some of the items listed may contain so little MSG that they pose no threat even to sensitive people. Others items listed can be eaten safely in moderation. However, because the amount of MSG in manufactured food is not labeled, how would you know?

Somewhat better information exists concerning the amount of MSG in natural foods. The table on page 92 may help you determine this amount, as I have listed them in order of increasing concentration of free glutamate or MSG. I have also included their content of MSG bound to protein that is not freely available for rapid absorption.

Remember that free glutamic acid is present in almost any food. You should be able to tolerate the small amounts present in such foods as chicken and duck at 44 and 69 mg/100 gm. Corn, tomatoes, and peas are probably okay at 130, 140, and 200 mg/100 gm except for the most sensitive MSG reactors. Even they should be able to eat them in small quantities, especially if they boil the corn and the peas well.

Natural Glutamate Content of Foods

Food	Bound Glutamate (mg/100 gm)	Free Glutamate (MSG) (mg/100 gm)
Cow's milk	819	2
Cod	2,101	9
Onions	208	18
Salmon	2,216	20
Human milk	229	22
Eggs	1,583	23
Pork	2,325	23
Beets	256	30
Green peppers	120	32
Beef	2,846	33
Carrots	218	33
Mackerel	2,382	36
Spinach	289	39
Chicken	3,309	44
Duck	3,636	69
Corn	1,765	130
Tomatoes	238	140
Peas	5,583	200
Parmesan cheese	9,847	1,200

Source: Modified from Institute of Food Technologists' Expert Panel on Food Safety and Nutrition, "Monosodium Glutamate." *Food Technology* 41, no. 5 (1987): 143–145.

Tomato products such as purées and sauces will concentrate the MSG present in tomatoes; these products may contain a high and symptom-stimulating MSG level. Cheeses such as Parmesan have naturally high levels, as we discussed.

Avoiding MSG Is Difficult

Add the many sources of MSG in natural foods to the many names found on the labels of manufactured food and you can see why avoiding MSG is difficult. How unfortunate that innocent-sounding names such as "natural flavoring" or "stock" on a label may hide MSG. Further difficulties arise because manufactured foods do not list the amount of MSG they contain.

As I am writing this book, we cannot even trust that a food labeled "no MSG added" is free of MSG. Manufacturers must admit to adding MSG only when it is added in its pure form. They can put a pound of MSG into a food and claim "no MSG added" if they use hydrolyzed protein, yeast extract, or other products with high levels of MSG. I understand that the FDA frowns on this practice, but I do not know if this prevents it from happening.

Until food manufacturers clearly identify all MSG in any form, my patients and you are stuck and will not be able to learn how much MSG they tolerate, nor can they select and eat foods with low MSG content.

To eat a low-MSG diet, you must consider the amount of MSG naturally present in food. Closely read labels, remembering all the clue words that can hide its presence. Do not buy foods that may contain too much MSG. If you buy and eat them, you take the chance of suffering uncomfortable and painful symptoms, symptoms that may even be dangerous.

In this country, with such heightened awareness of consumer protection, isn't this a terrible shame?

Guidelines to Discovering and Treating Food Allergy

It is a mistake to think that all patients are alike or that all allergic illnesses are the same.

Each patient is a special individual with a distinctive illness unlike any other patient's illness. For instance, food allergy contributes overwhelmingly to headache or wheezing for some patients; in others, food allergy contributes little. Some patients react badly to one food, while others tolerate that same food but suffer a severe reaction to another food. To keep food allergy in perspective, a medical caregiver must remember these differences in patients, illnesses, and causes. To do otherwise would be a great mistake.

There are certain guidelines I find helpful in putting food allergy in perspective. Let's look at these guidelines now.

No illness is allergy until it is diagnosed as such by your primary-care physician. Allergy does not cause all illness. You do not need an allergist to treat your headaches if a brain tumor causes them. You do not need skin testing for diarrhea if you suffer from bowel disease. Go to your medical care professional for diagnosis. Go to an allergist only after obtaining a proper primary diagnosis.

A nonallergic illness does not preclude allergy. This principle is not a contradiction of the first one. I treat many patients with brain lesions for the allergic component of their headaches, and I help patients with bowel inflammation alleviate the part of their cramps and diarrhea that is caused by allergy. They deserve the same care as any other patients with allergy.

Never ignore environmental allergy in diagnosing food allergy. It is best to assume that all patients react not only to the foods in their diet but also to the dust, mold, pollen, and pets in their environment. Patients both breathe and eat; to focus on one to the exclusion of the other means that the patient's illness will not be fully evaluated. I do not deny that I am often tempted to focus only on food allergy when investigating the allergic reactions of some patients—for example, the patients who react to a specific food (e.g., shrimp) in a specific way (e.g., hives). The obvious diagnosis is food allergy, solo and uncomplicated. Right?

Not necessarily. To understand this point, think of my patient as a bucket to which you are adding water. If the bucket is already full, any added water will slop over the side. If it's empty, you can add a lot of water before it spills over. In our analogy, the water that you add represents food allergy, and the water spilling over the side is the allergic reaction. Sometimes a patient's food allergy is superstrong and, just like adding water to a bucket filled to the brim will always cause it to overflow, eating the offending food will always lead to a reaction, all by itself.

At other times the food allergy is only moderately—or even mildly—strong, like a cup of water poured into a two-gallon bucket. The patient with this mild to moderate food allergy will not react to the food unless other allergies have "primed" him or her to react, just as the bucket must be almost full before a little extra water causes water to spill over the side.

This principle explains why food allergy so frequently strikes one day and not the next. On a particular day, sugar provokes a migraine; on another day, no headache. Perhaps on the day of the headache, the patient was exposed to a large amount of dust while cleaning out the basement plus a high ragweed pollen count on his or her afternoon walk. In this example, excess dust or ragweed exposure primed my patient for a headache brought on by sugar, a headache that would not occur on a day with low dust and ragweed exposure.

Environmental allergies such as allergy to dust, mold, and pollen often prime patients to react to foods. That's why categorizing any food allergy as "solo and uncomplicated" is frequently a mistake if environmental allergy is ignored. Foods often contribute only partially to symptoms, even in cases where the evidence seems to say that food alone is responsible.

Never ignore food allergy in diagnosing environmental allergy. This guideline goes hand in hand with the previous one. Just as we make a mistake when we ignore the influence of the environment on food allergy, we also make a mistake when we ignore the influence of foods on environmental allergy. Patients suffer if their medical care professionals err in either direction.

But what about the patient with solo, uncomplicated pollen allergy, the patient who sneezes only during the grass pollen season? Surely, foods do not cause this sneezing?

For an answer, let's return to thinking that the allergic patient must carry his or her allergies around in a bucket. For many, grass (or tree or ragweed) pollen allergy fills the bucket to overflowing. But does the overflow trickle out, or does it erupt in a flood? If the patient's bucket contains no other allergy, chances are it's a trickle. But if food allergy already partially fills the bucket, when trees, grass, or ragweed add their pollen, the overflow will gush out.

Similarly, my patients with pollen allergy can be far more comfortable if they avoid certain foods when the pollen count is high.

We see allergy to the food chemicals so commonly in our patients that my nurses and I routinely look for it when we investigate symptoms caused by pollen, dust, mold, and pet allergy. The single act of changing the diet during the time my patient suffers from something in the environment often determines whether we give our patients little help or pleasing relief. It can change a flood of allergy misery into a trickle of discomfort, a miserable pollen season into one that is merely uncomfortable.

Explore both food and environmental allergy in every patient. This guideline reinforces the previous two. A medical caregiver still serves his or her patient when he or she ignores food allergy while concentrating on environmental causes such as pollen, dust, mold, and pets. Ignoring the environment and concentrating on foods does the same. Breathing and eating are so basic to our existence that allergies encountered in either the air or the diet equally deteriorate our quality of life. Therefore we must pay attention to the influence of pollen, dust, and mold allergy on food allergy, and of food allergy on these environmental allergies. Only then can we treat our patients with the care they deserve.

Attack overpowering food allergy by attacking environmental allergy. In some cases a patient's food allergies are uncomplicated and easy to diagnose; avoidance of one or several foods solves the problem neatly. In other cases patients react to so many foods and suffer such devastating reactions that I feel almost powerless to help them.

Many examples spring to mind—patients with food allergy so universal that they suffer when eating or drinking practically every food or beverage in our modern diet. Some of the most tragic of these patients are those with bulimia or anorexia nervosa who also suffer from food allergy. Their horrendous food allergies make these formidable illnesses resistant to treatment.

The only effective way to treat these seemingly hopeless cases of food allergy is to eliminate as many nonfood allergens as possible. Using the analogy of the bucket, if the patient's food allergy causes it to overflow, the logical solution is to empty the bucket of any other allergic factors to make more room for food allergy. In other words, reduce the flood to a trickle.

In this approach to allergy care, the most important strategy is not the treatment of the food allergy itself but the aggressive treatment of any environmental allergy that may affect the patient, no matter how small. Amazingly, this works well.

Acidic foods, MSG, aspartic acid, and refined sugar are the most important food allergies. Although allergies to other foods, such as those to milk, wheat, or peanut butter, bother many people, the above-named food chemicals are more frequent causes of pain and discomfort.

Patients suffering allergic symptoms from diet chemicals need our help. There are many of these patients, part of an immense group of sufferers who react to chemicals in multiple foods. Diagnosing their symptoms can be baffling, treating the patients can be complicated, and the skills of an allergist sometimes are required. For these patients the potent and troubling food chemicals commonly cause illnesses, some directly and others indirectly. Treatment will fail unless these chemicals are recognized and reduced or eliminated. Only then can we help patients with their food allergies.

The prevalence of these food chemicals in our modern diet and their potential for provoking illness make it essential that allergic patients know how to find them. Not understanding their importance, where they hide in the diet, and how to avoid them condemns many patients to a life of pain and discomfort. This is so unnecessary.

Temper your diet with common sense. Some of our patients follow our dietary advice with religious fervor, never deviating; others take a more balanced approach, avoiding the excesses that bring on symptoms—and cheating at times. The latter are successfully treated. Compulsive followers eventually give up the diet because they find the strain of unswerving adherence too great.

In contrast, the patient who takes a more commonsense approach can stay on the diet for life, if necessary. When cheating brings the return of unpleasant symptoms, it reinforces the need to avoid the offending food and makes following the diet easier. This patient also should remain flexible—relax his or her vigilance as symptoms become less troubling.

For instance, if we treat environmental allergies aggressively with environmental corrections and allergy injections, the need for total avoidance decreases commensurately. Thus flexibility and common sense make the diet easier to follow.

Don't be discouraged. It is normal to feel discouraged when asked to eliminate foods and beverages you enjoy—and even crave. It takes a while to get used to the idea, but patients tell me that after about three years they usually forget they are following a diet.

It is often said that success breeds success, and it seems that when the diet has the desired effect of reducing or eliminating patients' symptoms, it is no longer an unacceptable burden. When we question patients about what they eat, my staff and I find they have no trouble avoiding the excessive sugar, MSG, low-calorie sweeteners, and acidic foods they once believed to be so essential. If you are similarly sensitive to these food chemicals, it can be the same for you.

I hope I have given you enough information to let you use the diet to diagnose your own possible sensitivity to these diet chemicals. If so, the following diet should help you.

The Adult and Child Allergy Elimination Diet

The diet I describe in this chapter is the same diet I ask our patients to follow after my nurses and I evaluate their symptoms and find evidence that they react to food chemicals. In this diet, we ask our patients to avoid certain foods and beverages while allowing them to eat others.

Food allergy frequently affects people who suffer from allergies, and most of our patients suffer from it to a greater or a lesser degree. You may also suffer from food allergy; if so, I want to help you discover which foods and beverages make you ill so that you can avoid them.

I designed this diet to help you learn about your food allergy. If you find that food chemicals trouble you, you can discover your allergy by following this diet. It will ease your discomfort, reduce food allergy's impact on your life, and help you feel well.

Many of my patients react to the food chemicals we examine in this diet. Each of these chemicals is made of substances normally present in our bodies and, when consumed in small quantities, causes no illness. However, our modern diet encourages excessive consumption of these chemicals. If you learn to avoid the foods and beverages that contain high levels of these chemicals, you remove their ability to hurt you.

The Food Chemicals

The food chemicals that concern us are (1) citric acid, which is commonly found in our diet, and less frequently encountered acids such as malic acid, tartaric acid, fumaric acid, and succinic acid; (2) refined sugar; (3) monosodium glutamate (MSG); and (4) aspartic acid, found in the artificial sweetener aspartame and sold under the brand names Equal and NutraSweet. The artificial sweetener saccharin, found in many products, also must be avoided.

Note: Citric acid also can be called citrate or citrus, malic acid can be called malate, tartaric acid can be called tartrate, fumaric acid can be called fumarate, and succinic acid can be called succinate.

Avoiding Chemicals in Your Foods and Beverages

The following foods and beverages contain large quantities of the above chemicals.

The acidic foods and beverages. You can tell which foods and drinks contain high levels of citric and related acids because you can taste the citrus or fruitiness. Many are natural foods—not processed or manufactured. For example, berries, cherries, grapes, and the citrus fruits—oranges, lemons, limes, and grapefruit—contain naturally high levels of citric acid.

Others are processed foods; a manufacturer adds citric or related acids to a beverage or a food to give it a pleasant, fruity taste. They always list this acid in the ingredients, so watch for the presence of citric acid, or less commonly, malic, tartaric, fumaric, or succinic acid. As mentioned, you may notice the acids labeled somewhat differently, with the –ic of citric replaced by –ate, as in sodium citrate or potassium citrate.

If the acid is high on the list of ingredients, the amount in the manufactured food is probably large, so you should avoid eating that product. If the acid is listed toward the end, it is probably present in small amounts and should not bother you. In all cases, let your sense of taste guide you; if it tastes fruity, leave it alone.

The following are some of the foods and beverages containing significant amounts of citric and other acids:

◇ candy, jam, jelly, preserves
◇ carbonated and noncarbonated beverages (soda pop, packaged drink mixes, etc.)
◇ desserts with a pronounced fruity taste (ice cream, flavored gelatin, pies, puddings, etc.)
◇ all fruits and berries listed below:

Apricots	Grapes	Plantains
Blackberries	Kiwis	Plums
Blueberries	Kumquats	Pomegranates
Cherries	Lemons	Prunes
Crab apples	Limes	Raisins
Cranberries	Loganberries	Raspberries
Currants	Mangoes	Rhubarb
Dates	Mulberries	Strawberries
Figs	Nectarines	Tangerines
Gooseberries	Oranges	
Grapefruit	Pineapples	

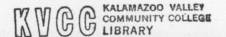

Also, any fruit juices or juice blends; tomatoes, tomato juice, and tomato-based products; and potatoes and potato products (potatoes are acid).

Refined sugar. Food manufacturers use refined sugar to sweeten many packaged foods and canned and bottled beverages. They always list it in the ingredients, although it may be under a name other than refined sugar: corn syrup, honey, brown sugar, molasses, maple syrup. All are refined sugars and can cause allergic symptoms. You need not pursue a diet completely free of all refined sugar; aim for a diet low enough in refined sugar that it does not set off your symptoms.

The following foods and beverages contain large amounts of refined sugar:

◇ candy, jam, jelly, preserves
◇ carbonated and noncarbonated beverages containing sugar
◇ desserts (cakes, cookies, ice cream, flavored gelatin, pies, sweet rolls, presweetened cereals, etc.)
◇ other products, including table sugar for coffee

Monosodium glutamate. High quantities of monosodium glutamate are naturally present in foods such as mushrooms, kelp (seaweed), and scallops. Do not eat them. Food manufacturers use MSG to flavor prepared meats such as breakfast sausages, bratwurst, hot dogs, luncheon meats, pot pies, frozen prepared entrées, and TV dinners. MSG gives these foods an extra-hearty taste that brings pleasure to the palate but distressing symptoms to many allergy sufferers. Do not eat them.

Watch for MSG in soups and breaded products; look for it in many snack foods such as crackers, chips, and nuts. Check for it if you eat at Oriental restaurants; usually you can avoid it by asking the cook to prepare the meal without monosodium glutamate. As fermentation releases large quantities of MSG, expect to find it in fermented products such as cheese, soy sauce, and alcoholic beverages; avoid them.

To determine whether processed foods contain MSG, look for it on the label. If you see it listed, do not buy the product. Sometimes MSG hides under a number of names, including autolyzed yeast extract, dried yeast and yeast nutrients, calcium or sodium caseinate, textured and whey protein and protein hydrolyzate or hydrolyzed vegetable/plant protein (contains 10 to 40% MSG). It may even hide under the catchall phrase "natural flavors"; short of writing to the manufacturer to ask if the "natural flavors" include MSG, you do not know whether the food contains MSG. The safest solution is not to buy these products.

Artificial sweeteners. You commonly find aspartame (NutraSweet and Equal) and saccharin in carbonated and noncarbonated diet beverages, diet foods, and low-calorie sweeteners for home use. Do not use them while you follow this diet.

Using the Diet

Now that you know the food chemicals you should avoid, we will look at the foods you can eat while following the diet. The following thoughts will help guide you as you follow the elimination diet.

What to watch for. While you follow the diet you will be watching to see if eliminating certain foods and beverages relieves your symptoms. These symptoms may include a stuffy nose, headaches, hives, asthma, abdominal pains, diarrhea, or any of the numerous other pains and discomforts that plague the allergic patient. Watch for relief from these symptoms as you follow the diet.

During the diet. How you start the diet depends on how often you suffer symptoms. If your symptoms occur frequently—daily or several times a week—avoid the above foods and beverages for two weeks to allow you to determine if they worsen your symptoms.

If your symptoms occur less frequently—weeks or months apart—you may not learn anything from two weeks of elimination, even if you follow the diet meticulously. If you are symptom-free, you could not tell if the diet worked or if you simply didn't experience any symptoms during the two weeks you followed it. Therefore, when your symptoms return infrequently, you need not completely abstain from these foods and beverages; instead, reduce their use. If symptoms strike, recall the foods and beverages you consumed in the previous twenty-four hours; you may be able to identify the foods and beverages that contributed to your symptoms. Usually they are the foods and beverages listed above.

If your symptoms appear only during one season or at a special time of the year, you will need to follow this diet during that season or time only. You may eat these foods without trouble at other times.

Testing the diet. Take a second step to make sure the particular foods and beverages you eliminated actually cause your discomfort. Return them to your diet; if your symptoms flare on reintroduction, you will be more confident that they cause your symptoms. How you reintroduce these foods is up to you. You can return all of them at once in large quantities to see if they provoke your symptoms. Alternatively, you may decide to cautiously return these foods and beverages to your diet, first reintroducing the foods and beverages you miss the most, adding them back carefully in small quantities. In this cautious approach, you would continue to add foods and beverages until you started to experience the symptoms lessened by the diet. Adding one food at a time probably will not help you; your pain and discomfort are caused by the total quantity of all these foods and beverages in your daily diet.

Living with the diet. As you become accustomed to this diet, you will find that you can eat and drink many of the prohibited foods and beverages if you limit the quantities to a level you can tolerate. For instance, you may comfortably eat one or two cookies in a day, but not ten. You may tolerate a little ketchup, but not a glass of tomato juice. You may tolerate some cheese, but probably not as much as you would like. Eventually you should be able to determine your level of tolerance for these foods and beverages, making the diet less onerous and you more comfortable.

What You Can Eat

The following meal lists contain foods that my patients usually can eat and drink comfortably. To help you plan your menus, I listed some name brands of products that I believe are low in the chemicals that trouble my patients. Because ingredients in products can change, be sure to read the label before eating these products.

Breakfast

Cereals (use any of the following with milk)

Cheerios	Puffed Rice
Cream of Rice	Puffed Wheat
Cream of Wheat	Rice Krispies
Grape-Nuts Flakes	Shredded Wheat
Malt-O-Meal	Wheat Chex
Oatmeal	

Eggs

Bacon, ham

Toast with butter or margarine

Lunch

Grain products (may be used at any meal):

Baking powder biscuits	Flour tortillas
Breads (rye, wheat, rice)	Muffins (banana, bran, free of
Crackers (without MSG)	citric acid and low in sugar)
Croissants (plain)	Noodles and macaroni
Flat breads	

Rice (white rice, wild rice, rice cakes)

The following are lunch suggestions:

◇ Sandwich with beef, pork, fish, or fowl. Bread may be spread with butter or margarine; garnish with lettuce or a pickle.

◇ Salad with oil and vinegar (not wine vinegar), olive oil, or mayonnaise without lemon juice, citrus, or MSG added. Lettuce, spinach, onions, carrots, cucumbers, radishes, olives, celery. Accompany with any of the allowed fruits.

◇ Sausage, hamburgers, or hot dogs are allowed if free of MSG.

Dinner

Meat (beef, pork, fish, fowl)
Salad (same as lunch salad)
Grain products (same as for lunch)
Vegetables (any of the following):

Artichokes	Celery
Asparagus	Okra
Beets	Olives (without pimento)
Boiled broccoli	Parsnips
Boiled cabbage	Radishes
Boiled corn	Rutabaga
Boiled green beans	Squash
Carrots	Turnips

Fruits—you may have two or more servings of:

Apples	Peaches
Bananas	Pears
Cantaloupe	Watermelon
Muskmelon	

Beverages

Coffee	Unflavored bottled water
Milk	Water
Tea	

Snacks

Any crackers or pretzels processed without MSG, sugar, or acids
Any nuts without additives other than salt:

Almonds	Macadamia nuts
Brazil nuts	Pecans
Cashews	Pistachios
Filberts	Sunflower seeds
Hazelnuts	Walnuts

Acceptable Foods by Food Group

The following is a list of some of the foods that you can eat while you follow my diet. I have classified the foods according to biologic relationship with examples for each group. If you have a strong allergy to any of these foods (e.g., nuts or fish), you must avoid it—do not use it in the diet. If you have a weak allergy to some of the foods I list as acceptable, continue to use these foods unless they cause symptoms. Sometimes you can eat them one or two days out of three (rotating foods) without suffering symptoms.

Animal Groups

Amphibians: frogs

Crustaceans: crabs, lobsters, shrimp

Eggs

Fish: bass, cod, crappie, flounder, haddock, halibut, salmon, scrod, sunfish, trout, tuna, walleye, whitefish

Fowl: chicken, Cornish game hen, duck, goose, turkey

Milk products: butter, milk casein (cheese product)

Mollusks: abalone, clams, oysters, snails

Red-meat animals: beef, lamb, mutton, pork, veal (roasts, steaks, chops), bacon, ham

Plant Groups

Beech family: beechnut, chestnut

Birch family: filbert, hazelnut

Cashew family: cashew, pistachio

Ginger family: cardamom, ginger

Goosefoot family: beet, spinach, Swiss chard

Gourd family: cantaloupe (muskmelon), casaba, cucumber, honeydew melon, pumpkin, squash, watermelon

Grass family: barley, oats, rice, rye, wheat

Laurel family: avocado, bay leaf, cinnamon

Lecythis: Brazil nut

Lily family: asparagus, chives, garlic, leek, onion

Madder family: cottonseed, okra

Mint family: basil, Japanese artichoke, marjoram, mint, oregano, peppermint, sage, savory, spearmint, thyme

Morning glory family: sweet potato, yam

Mustard family: radish, rutabaga, turnip

Myrtle family: allspice

Olive family: olive

Parsley family: caraway, carrot, celeriac, celery, dill, parsley

Pepper family: black pepper

Plum family: almond

Poppy family: poppy seed

Sunflower family: artichoke, Jerusalem artichoke, lettuce, sunflower

Tea family: tea

Walnut family: black walnut, butternut, English hickory nut, pecan

Additional Information

Fruits. Most of our patients are able to tolerate two or three servings of the recommended fruits, including apples, bananas, cantaloupe, muskmelon, peaches, pears, and watermelon. These fruits are lower in acid; avoid the rest.

Cheese. Many of our patients tolerate only a limited amount of cheese, if any at all. Cheese contains MSG; the more aged the cheese, the more MSG it contains.

Legumes. Sensitivity to this food category, which includes beans, peas, peanuts, and soybeans, varies; you may or may not be able to tolerate them. Storing fresh peas and beans for twenty-four hours before preparing them, boiling them well, and discarding the boiled water help reduce symptoms in many patients.

Potatoes. Potatoes are a special problem. Most of our patients tolerate only a few servings of potatoes per week; others cannot tolerate any potatoes. Use caution and watch your symptoms when you include them in your diet. Boiling them well may be the best way to serve them.

Corn and corn products. Be careful. Many of our patients—perhaps 50 percent—react to corn, especially popcorn or corn on the cob. Use caution and watch for symptoms when eating corn products. Cutting corn free from the cob and boiling it well help many patients tolerate it.

Cabbage family. Many patients react poorly to raw cabbage, broccoli, Brussels sprouts, and cauliflower but can eat them when boiled until soft.

Refined sugar. Tolerated in small to moderate quantities by many of our patients. While following the two-week elimination diet, eat no refined sugar. After you finish the two weeks, you can start to use some sugar. If you are mildly or moderately sensitive, you should find that you tolerate a little honey on bread, a small slice of cake, several cookies, a doughnut or sweet roll, a little soda, or a teaspoon of sugar in your coffee once a day.

Keep the total amount of refined sugar or honey consumed in a day to the quantity you tolerate. If you crave sugar, you may not be able to include even a small amount in your diet.

Vinegar. Do not use either wine or apple cider vinegar. Use only vinegar made from grain and as small an amount as possible.

Vitamins and food supplements. Stop taking all vitamins and food supplements during the two-week trial elimination period. Many supplements contain aspartic and glutamic acid (MSG). In other supplements the protein has been hydrolyzed to amino acids, freeing glutamic (MSG) and aspartic acid to be absorbed quickly. Vitamin C may be combined with citric acid to prevent deterioration.

Alcohol. No alcohol should be consumed during the two-week trial elimination.

Living with the Diet

We followed the evolution of a diet that reduces or eliminates the foods and beverages that most commonly cause this widespread affliction. With this knowledge you can now find relief from pain and discomfort by carefully choosing the foods you eat and the beverages you drink. You can identify the allergies that torment you; you need no longer tolerate this suffering. You can look forward to each day, expecting to feel well.

Now you must use this information to change your diet so that you can reach your precious goal of good health.

In the next few sections, I will help you do this. I will tell you how to apply the information you have learned while you shop for food, prepare meals to eat at home, and select foods from the menu when eating in a restaurant.

How strictly you need to follow my suggestions depends on your degree of sensitivity to the food chemicals. It also depends on whether (1) you are following the two-week elimination diet or (2) you have completed the two-week diet and are returning these foods to your diet.

A word of caution: I am a specialist only in the allergic illnesses, including food allergy. I am not a specialist in low-cholesterol, diabetic, or other diets. If you have a medical condition that requires you to follow a special diet, you may not be able to eat some of the foods I recommend. To obtain help in adapting this elimination diet to your needs, consult your medical care professional, a dietitian, or both.

Reading Labels

The magnitude of the lifestyle change made necessary by this food elimination diet becomes apparent while you read the labels on the groceries in your kitchen cabinets. You probably will find that the foods and beverages there are filled with refined sugar, MSG, citric acids, or low-calorie sweeteners.

As you read these labels, you will realize that one of the first things you must change is your shopping habits. You can no longer grab the old familiar products from the grocery shelves; you must avoid many of your old favorites. You must select foods with small amounts of or no MSG, citric acid, refined sugar, or low-calorie sweeteners.

The Importance of the Label

While we find it easy to identify natural foods that contain large amounts of the food chemicals we are avoiding, such as tomatoes and citrus fruits, we find it much harder to identify these chemicals in prepared food products. And these prepackaged foods frequently contain troublesome amounts of food chemicals. That's why we must learn to read food labels—they tell us which foods to buy and which foods to avoid.

The Food and Drug Administration requires food manufacturers to list the ingredients used in the foods they produce. Manufacturers list these ingredients in descending order according to the amount the product contains; they list the ingredient present in the largest amount first. Then they list the ingredient present in the second-largest amount, and so on, until all of the ingredients are listed according to the quantity in or used to prepare the food.

Food-sensitive people find this list of ingredients a valuable guide. Reading the label allows them to avoid the foods that cause unacceptable symptoms. This amount varies from patient to patient.

Some of my patients find that they tolerate certain chemicals such as sugar and the fruit acids only if the quantity in the food is small. They can recognize a product with small quantities because the foods will not taste overly sweet or extra fruity and the sugar or acid will be listed near the end of the list of ingredients. Therefore, if an ingredient such as sugar or citric acid is listed far down the list of ingredients, the food may be acceptable even if your tolerance is small.

Some of my patients similarly tolerate any amount of MSG and low-calorie sweeteners; others can tolerate small amounts, and some cannot tolerate even minute quantities. These latter supersensitive patients must avoid all foods containing MSG and low-calorie sweeteners, along with foods with pronounced sweet or fruity flavors.

Some Examples of Labels

To illustrate the various terms used by food manufacturers, I have reproduced the lists of ingredients for several prepackaged foods. When the list of ingredients contains chemicals that my patients poorly tolerate, they are indicated in bold-face type to call your attention to them. Food allergy patients should avoid eating foods with these ingredients. If I did not highlight any ingredients, eating this food should not cause any symptoms.

Spaghetti Noodles
Ingredients: semolina, niacinamide, ferrous sulfate (iron), thiamine mononitrate, and riboflavin.

Note: Contains no problem ingredients.

Complete Buttermilk Pancake Mix
Ingredients: bleached enriched flour (bleached flour, malted barley flour, niacin, iron, thiamine, mononitrate [vitamin B$_1$], riboflavin [vitamin B$_2$]), yellow corn flour, **sugar, dextrose,** baking powder (baking soda, monocalcium phosphate, sodium aluminum phosphate), buttermilk, salt, egg whites, mono- and diglycerides, nonfat milk, lecithin, eggs, hydrogenated soybean oil, **corn syrup solids.**

The various forms of sugar have been highlighted in the pancake mix ingredient list. Refined sugar can be a problem for many people if it is consumed in too large a quantity. Remember, in listing the quantity of a food chemical, ingredients are listed in descending order of content, with the ingredient accounting for the highest percentage of the total product listed first.

In the ingredient list above, sugar is the third ingredient listed, dextrose is the fourth, and another form of sugar—corn syrup solids—ends the list. Although the label does not tell us what percentage of the total content these sugars represent, this mix probably contains too much sugar for patients on our diet. If the item tastes sweet, you should not eat it during the two-week elimination diet. No matter where it is listed in the ingredient list, the sugar content is probably too high.

Skillet Hamburger Mix
Ingredients: enriched macaroni, vegetable shortening (contains one or both of the following partially hydrogenated oils: soybean, cottonseed), **cheddar cheese** (milk, salt, cheese cultures, enzymes, color added), corn starch, **tomato** (with color protected by sodium bisulfite), buttermilk, salt, **sugar, hydrolyzed vegetable protein,** onion, **corn syrup,** disodium phosphate (for smooth sauce), garlic, **natural flavors, sodium caseinate** (a milk protein), citric acid (for flavor), dipotassium phosphate (for smooth sauce), Yellow No. 5, and Yellow No. 6.

Don't use this mix. Not only does it contain MSG in the form of cheese, tomato, hydrolyzed vegetable protein, and natural flavors (MSG), but also sugar, corn syrup (refined sugar), and citric acid (tomato is also acid). In addition, it contains sodium caseinate, made by precipitating casein from skim milk by the addition of an acid and yielding an MSG-enriched flavoring. In the diet it can cause the same problems as cheese and other MSG sources. This product contains too many ingredients that are troublesome. Do not buy it.

Chicken Coating Mix

Ingredients: bleached bromated wheat flour, **dextrin** (from corn), partially hydrogenated soybean and cottonseed oils, salt, paprika, **malted barley,** spices (mustard flour, celery seed, chili pepper, black pepper, thyme, basil, red pepper, cloves, oregano, rosemary), **sugar, yeast,** beet powder (for color), garlic powder, onion powder, **natural hickory smoke flavor,** TBHQ, and calcium propionate (to preserve freshness).

This coating mix may contain MSG in the natural hickory smoke flavor, malted barley, and yeast. It does contain sugars. If you use it, you may experience discomfort, especially if MSG is present and if other poorly tolerated foods are consumed within the surrounding day or two. Think twice about buying it.

Canned Meat

Ingredients: chopped pork shoulder meat with ham meat added and salt, water, **sugar,** and sodium nitrate.

Note: This meat product contains no problem ingredients other than sugar, which should be in too small a quantity to bother you.

Chicken Flavor Rice Mix

Ingredients: enriched egg white macaroni product, **natural flavors,** salt, partially hydrogenated vegetable oil (soybean and/or cottonseed), food starch, **modified corn syrup, sugar,** chicken, **monosodium glutamate,** onions, modified vegetable gum, **sodium caseinate,** garlic, **yeast, chicken broth,** soy flour, parsley, spice, disodium inosinate, disodium guanylate.

Hydrogenated vegetable oil is okay in our elimination diet. Other ingredients are not. This mix contains modified corn syrup (sugar), sugars, and MSG (as monosodium glutamate, sodium caseinate and possibly as "yeast," "natural flavors," and "chicken broth"). The combination of these chemicals can make you suffer. Do not buy this product.

Gelatin Dessert
Ingredients: **sugar, gelatin,** adipic acid (for tartness), disodium phosphate (controls acidity), **fumaric acid** (for tartness), artificial color, artificial flavor.

Note: This product is probably too sweet and too acid. Gelatin, depending on its preparation, may contain MSG. Leave it on the shelf.

Instant Pudding
Ingredients: **sugar, dextrose** (corn sugar), corn starch modified, sodium phosphates (for proper set), salt, hydrogenated soybean oil with BHA (preservative), di- and monoglycerides (to prevent foaming), nonfat milk, artificial color (including Yellow No. 5 and Yellow No. 6), artificial and **natural flavor.**

Note: Contains too much sugar and that mysterious term "natural flavor," which may be MSG. Do not buy it.

Tuna in Spring Water
Ingredients: chunk light tuna in spring water, vegetable broth, salt, **hydrolyzed protein.**

Note: Contains MSG; don't use this product. Why do so many tuna preparations contain MSG?

Fruit Juice
Ingredients: **grape, apple, and passion fruit juices** from concentrates, **natural flavor,** vitamin C.

Note: Natural flavor—MSG? This product is also probably too acid. Don't use it.

Pear Halves in Heavy Syrup
Ingredients: pears, water, **corn syrup.**

Note: Pears are low-acid fruit—use them, but first rinse the syrup off thoroughly with clear water.

If you feel that label reading is just too complicated for you, do not despair. You will develop this skill over time. If you eat or drink something that causes you to experience symptoms, check the label; the product may contain a chemical not acceptable on the elimination diet. As you learn to recognize the problematic food additives and chemicals by name, you will find it easier to avoid buying the products that contain them.

Is This Too Much to Expect?

Do our patients find that they can change their shopping habits? Yes, they do. Do they find the sacrifices they make—eliminating favorite foods and beverages—more than they can stand? Not when they begin to feel better. They follow the diet because they are not quitters. They prove their determination to find their way to health by refusing to accept their illness as some force they cannot conquer, some mystery they cannot understand, or some sickness they cannot treat.

By coming to our office for treatment, they demonstrate their commitment to do what must be done to understand and overcome their illness. Like so many patients before them, they tolerate a wrenching diet change to free themselves of pain and discomfort, bloating and achiness, melancholy and tiredness, so they can live normally.

Shopping for Groceries

Checking the ingredients of every item we might purchase makes grocery shopping more complicated. When we recommend this complicated task to our patients they often ask, "Exactly how should I select foods at the store?" I decided that the best way to answer this question was to put myself in their place, so I made a trip to the grocery store.

Since I share my patients' food sensitivity and must continually examine the foods and beverages I buy, I found it easy to imagine my patients' problems while I shopped.

Cereals

As I push my cart through the door of the grocery store, I enter the cereal section, with its confusing array of brightly colored boxes.

Ignoring the sugar-coated cereals for obvious reasons, I examine the rest. One after another, I read the lists of ingredients. On many of the uncoated cereals, sugar is listed as the second or third ingredient—and some list two or even three types of refined sugar under such names as brown sugar, corn syrup, honey, and so on. My sugar-sensitive patients would tolerate these cereals poorly.

It is only later, in a less prominent part of the store, that I find the low-sugar cereals my food allergy patients can tolerate—the Puffed Rice, Puffed Wheat, Rice Krispies, and Shredded Wheat. Also in this section are the boxes of Cream of Wheat and plain oatmeal that I eat (flavored oatmeal may contain sugar and citrus).

If you select cereals with a delicious, sweet taste, you will undoubtedly have selected those with a high sugar content. If you select cereals with a refreshing fruity taste, you will have selected those with high amounts of citric, malic, and/or fumaric acids.

I do not mean to say that flavored cereals are not nutritious foods and perfectly good to eat. What I am saying is that they are fine to eat unless the fruit flavorings cause noses to stuff up or skin to itch and break out in large, red, blotchy hives. A breakfast of high-sugar cereal is fine unless it causes throats to hurt, voices to turn raspy, or breathing to become labored.

The point I want to emphasize is that although these cereals taste delightful, the enjoyment they bring the food-chemical-sensitive person may not outweigh the resulting aggravating symptoms.

The Fruit Section

Next I enter the fruit section of the store. In the citrus display, the oranges and grapefruit radiate an irresistible attractiveness, tempting me to buy and enjoy them. However, if I do, the acid factory in my stomach would go on overtime, sending its hydrochloric acid burning painfully down my intestines and up my esophagus. Regretfully, I must pass by these handsome fruits.

Thankfully, you and I can eat many lower-acid fruits on our diet. The muskmelons and watermelons look equally inviting and delicious. The bananas almost glow with ripeness, and the bright red apples looked as healthy as the blush on the cheek of a child playing in the winter snow. The pears are full and ripe, the peaches swollen with juice.

Why are apples and pears so well tolerated by my patients? Both contain lots of malic acid. My patients' experiences suggest that malic acid is better tolerated than the other fruit-derived acids, especially citric and tartaric. They can eat and drink more malic acid before they start to suffer.

The Vegetable Section

Patients following our diet should find selecting vegetables easier than selecting fruits, with the exception of the nightshade family of vegetables. The tomatoes, potatoes, eggplant, and red and green peppers that make up this family carry too high a content of MSG and citric acid, so these vegetables must be avoided.

I find it especially hard to tell my chemical-sensitive patients that they must give up potatoes; so many of us are accustomed to including them with our meals almost daily. Fortunately, rice and pasta make good substitutes for this nutritious but troubling food.

As I proceed through the vegetable section, I spot many acceptable salad ingredients. All varieties of lettuce and spinach are tolerated, as well as carrots, celery, radishes, and onions. Mixed with sunflower seeds and ripe olives, these vegetables make a tasty salad, wholesome and nutritious. Unfortunately, I am still unsure what salad dressing to advise (that's why I eat my salad without dressing). Olive oil is all right. Grain-based or white vinegar and oil dressing is probably acceptable for those who cannot eat salad without dressing. But salad dressings loaded with tomato, citrus, fruit juice, and sugar are not acceptable.

While I'm on the subject of salads, a word of warning: Be cautious of croutons. Although they add a gratifying crunchiness to a salad, many brands contain MSG in one of its many names or disguises, such as dried cheese or hydrolyzed vegetable protein, and can trouble my MSG-sensitive patients. If you make your own, you can avoid this flavoring.

As I continue through the vegetable section, I come to the cabbage family display. Solid, leafy green heads of cabbage nestle together, near darker green Brussels sprouts that so resemble their larger relatives. Cauliflower look like snow-white flowers snipped from their stems, with broccoli looking like bouquets of flowers picked before they opened. Each of these vegetables contributes valuable nutrition to a meal. Many of my patients can eat vegetables of the cabbage family either raw or cooked, but some suffer symptoms if they eat them raw and must either avoid them or boil them well before eating.

Later, in the freezer section, I see many vegetable selections that are acceptable for food-sensitive patients—fresh frozen peas, beans, corn, carrots, broccoli, cauliflower, and onions in various combinations. Most of my patients tolerate these frozen vegetables; those with minor sensitivity can serve them steamed, but those who are more sensitive will need to boil them well or avoid them altogether. Avoid mixtures containing green and red peppers and mushrooms, unless present in small amounts.

I pass by the selections of frozen vegetables in sauce without stopping. Food manufacturers often add MSG, cheese, or refined sugar to sauces to make them taste pleasing, and although many people tolerate these flavoring agents well, my food-chemical-sensitive patients tolerate them poorly.

Regretfully, I also pass by a food I love to eat—corn on the cob. I don't know what divine purpose is served by instilling in us an overpowering craving for the foods that cause us pain. I do know that since many of my patients and I crave this delicious late-summer treat but experience bloating and abdominal discomfort when we eat it, we had best stick to corn cut from the cob and boiled until soft. Or boil the corn on the cob until the kernels are mushy-soft and hope you can tolerate it.

Many other vegetables may be acceptable for patients on our diet—vegetables I have not learned to eat and thus do not fully appreciate. If my patients know they eat them without symptoms, they can include them in their diets.

The Meat Section

Unprocessed meat (plain meat without added flavorings). For food allergy sufferers, beef, pork, lamb, chicken, turkey, and fish are godsends because most patients tolerate them well. Unfortunately, a few unlucky souls show a positive skin test to these meats and tolerate them poorly. Sometimes fish allergy can be not only troubling but also downright dangerous. In general, though, my patients should tolerate foods in this section.

Which meats can the food-sensitive person purchase? Any of the unprocessed cuts of beef, such as roasts or steaks, can be chosen. Thinly sliced roast beef for sandwiches probably is acceptable, as long as the preparation did not include a marinade that contains MSG, such as wine or soy sauce. Avoid steak sauce, as it is likely to contain poorly tolerated ingredients.

Unprocessed pork chops, roasts, and bacon are acceptable, as well as lamb for those who enjoy its flavor. Fish is superb.

For food-sensitive patients, chicken is a great food. I often grill a large number of chicken legs and breasts and then freeze them so I can reheat them in a microwave for quick lunches and dinners. Seasoned with a little salt and pepper, they make a delicious meal free of troublesome flavorings.

Turkey also is an excellent food for my patients, but they must be careful when purchasing whole turkeys. Many are injected with an MSG-containing flavoring, often hydrolyzed vegetable protein. MSG-sensitive persons must avoid them.

Processed meat (meat to which flavoring has been added). Here is the section of the grocery store most likely to frustrate my patients—sandwich meats, breakfast sausages, processed lunch and dinner meats, breaded-meat selections, and processed meat in sauces. These are such a convenience for the busy person—just heat and serve for a meal, or fold into a sandwich to eat at work or at school. What could be easier?

It's not easy to find processed meat that won't cause headaches or diarrhea in food-chemical-sensitive people. It can be a real time-waster—reading label after label searching for meat preparations that are free of MSG, excess sugar, and the citric acids. Not many are available.

In processed meats, the most important food chemical to avoid is MSG in all its forms. As I hunt through the selections, I find label after label listing MSG, autolyzed yeast, and hydrolyzed vegetable protein (one label called it hydrolyzed plant protein, a novel way to describe MSG).

Many labels list "natural flavorings," and because natural flavorings may contain MSG, and because MSG is likely to be used for its ability to enhance the flavor in meat preparations, I consider all selections in the processed-meat section to contain MSG if they contain natural flavorings. I do not buy them.

Although most of my food-chemical-sensitive patients tolerate the small amounts of sugar and citrus found in meats, they tolerate MSG poorly—even in small quantities. For them, having to avoid MSG makes shopping in the processed-meat section a real pain.

I find shopping for processed meat easier if I find a few products that are free of MSG and excess sugar and buy only these products. Fortunately, a brand of sandwich meats has many acceptable products—Louis Rich. I find the turkey preparations delicious, especially the smoked turkey ham and turkey nuggets. On this trip I noticed another acceptable brand, Mr. Turkey, which advertises on the label that it is free of MSG. The labels on both Mr. Turkey and most of the Louis Rich products do not list any suspicious ingredients, including "natural flavorings." Both contain sugar, but I think the amount is small and should be acceptable.

I enjoy the flavor of bratwurst, but I couldn't find any acceptable varieties on this trip. This was not a major inconvenience because I know of a grocery store that makes its own bratwurst, and the butcher insists it is free of MSG and MSG-containing flavorings. Since I have eaten it without experiencing any bloating or abdominal pain, I believe him.

After checking the labels on many breakfast sausages, I found two brands that are clearly acceptable: Jones Dairy Farm Little Pork Sausages, and Woodend Pork Sausage and Pork Sausage Links. Since breakfast sausages make breakfast a more enjoyable meal, finding these two brands was a real triumph.

In buying any food, including meat, remember: Always read the labels, as ingredients can change.

The Dairy Section

Choices are relatively simple in the dairy section. Butter and fresh milk are acceptable. Sweet-tasting products, including ice cream, are not—they contain refined sugar and may contain MSG and one of the citrus acids. Because it is a fermented product, and because fermentation releases MSG, cheese must be approached with caution. The longer a cheese is aged, the more MSG is released, so some of the aged cheeses have large amounts of MSG.

Between fresh milk and aged cheese there is room for compromise. Less sensitive patients (those with milder and less frequent symptoms) may tolerate minimally aged cheese products such as American processed cheese or cottage cheese if they do not eat too much. Always read the list of ingredients first. Since cheesemakers do not list the amount of MSG formed naturally during cheese manufacturing, eating these cheeses is always chancy.

Some brands of plain, unflavored yogurt may be fermented less than others and may be acceptable in moderate amounts for those who consider yogurt important. I advise my yogurt-loving patients to buy several brands and experiment.

Soups

I enjoy soup, but I have had difficulty finding one without MSG. They are scarce. During my shopping trip I noticed that the label on one brand of soup read "No MSG." Great, I thought. Finally, a soup I can eat. No such luck! The label listed several varieties of aged cheese as well as that warning sign "natural flavoring." Although the manufacturer did not add pure MSG to the soup, it was added in the form of cheese and perhaps also in the natural flavoring.

I wonder whether food manufacturers know that aged cheese is one of the richest sources of MSG found in foods. They should; they have access to knowledgeable food scientists. What other reason might they have for adding aged cheese to soup and then proudly claiming it is free of MSG?

This experience prompts me to repeat the three most important shopping instructions for the food-sensitive person: (1) read the label, (2) read the label, and (3) read the label.

Reflections on Shopping

I found choosing foods without MSG, low-calorie sweeteners, excess citrus acids, and excess refined sugar an effort, but it can be done. I do it, and my patients do it. The important thing is not to lose sight of the benefits—patients sensitive to food feel much better if they choose foods they can eat without pain and discomfort.

Remember, always read the label. Food manufacturers can—and do—change ingredients. Sitting in my freezer are two pork sausage preparations that used to be free of MSG. They now contain it, but I didn't read the labels of these safe foods when I bought them. I won't eat them. I should have followed my own advice and read the labels.

As I shopped, I was troubled by the many foods that contain small amounts of refined sugar, even some of the foods I have recommended. Remember a famous saying about government spending: "A billion dollars here, a billion dollars there, and soon you are talking about real money." Food allergy is like that. A little sugar here, a little sugar there, and soon my patients are talking about headaches, hives, stuffy noses, and all kinds of other allergy miseries. Watch the sugar, even the small amounts. If you can, choose foods without any refined sugar.

I did not cover all the food choices my patients face when they shop; many are discussed elsewhere, including in the section on snacking. Nor have I covered all the acceptable food selections—just those I examined on my trip through the grocery store. My purpose was not to tell you what to buy; I wanted to tell you *how* to shop. I hope I have provided some helpful ideas for shopping wisely.

You should understand that you have the power to change the way food is prepared—far more power than anything I possess from my lectures and writing. By buying brands such as Louis Rich, Mr. Turkey, Jones Dairy Farm, and Woodend, and leaving products with MSG and "natural flavoring" on the shelf, you will be sending a clear message to food manufacturers. The law of supply and demand will force manufacturers to provide more products that food-allergy patients will buy.

Eating at Home

In the previous section, I presented some thoughts on shopping. We looked for foods that do not contain the dietary chemicals my patients must limit or avoid entirely. In this section, I want to share some ideas on how to prepare everyday meals at home, using foods low in acid, refined sugar, MSG, and low-calorie sweeteners.

How I Follow the Diet at Home

Being forced to follow the same advice my patients must follow gives me a unique perspective on how to prepare meals while following our diet. I know acceptable meals can be prepared because I prepare them. Each day the diet guides my food and beverage choices.

If you suffer these chemical sensitivities, I hope my experiences help you plan your diet. Please understand that as I describe my diet, I am not including all the foods and beverages that can be used, just those I usually eat and drink.

Breakfast

If there ever was a creature of habit, it is I. For some unknown reason, my stomach wakes me at about five o'clock every morning, telling me to rise and shine—it's hungry! My breakfast certainly shows this same love of habit—I eat the same thing almost every day. Into a small pan goes water, a cup of oatmeal, a little salt, and a sliced banana—stirred until the oatmeal thickens. A banana may not seem sweet to someone whose diet includes lots of refined sugar, but for me and for others who must avoid refined sugar, the taste of a banana mixed with hot oatmeal is like the finest sweet treat. With a serving of skim milk, I have a breakfast I enjoy.

Unfortunately, not all my patients can eat the same meal every day. We treat many patients allergic to many foods. Fortunately for these unlucky people, if they change their diet frequently (rotate their foods), they can eat without discomfort because eating a wide variety of foods reduces the impact of any one food that may cause symptoms. For them it would be a mistake to eat oatmeal every day, as I do. They can rotate oatmeal with Cream of Wheat, Puffed Rice, Shredded Wheat, or other fine cereals low in sugar and without low-calorie sweeteners or citrus.

I confess that I do not eat oatmeal every day. Once or twice a week, usually on the weekend, I enjoy a delightful breakfast of bacon or sausages with sunny-side-up eggs and pancakes or toast with apple butter. I thoroughly enjoy this meal.

However, if you eat these foods for breakfast, be careful of several important items. Make sure the sausage is free of MSG in all of its varied names, such as hydrolyzed vegetable protein, autolyzed yeast extract, or natural flavoring. If you eat pancakes, try to find preparations with little refined sugar. Do not use syrup on the pancakes—a little salt or butter or an egg on top of the pancakes will have to serve as your syrup.

Do not overdo the apple butter (although I think this spread is better tolerated than the high-sugar or high-citrus jellies and jams). Also, forget the fruit juice; it concentrates the fruit's acid.

Lunch

Lunch is not a particularly difficult meal to prepare while following my diet. In my case, I ensure an acceptable meal by my habit of taking a brown-bag lunch to the office each day.

I usually eat the same lunch—whole-grain bread plus lettuce and meat, usually turkey breast or other prepared meats made from turkey—which is fine with me. There is no reason not to use beef- or pork-based sliced meat; many are now prepared without MSG-containing flavorings. To find these sandwich meats, spend time reading the list of ingredients on the sandwich meats at your local grocery; there are selections you can use. This is a great improvement over the few selections available when I started to realize the importance of food allergy and discovered that the hunt for acceptable sandwich meats without MSG flavoring constituted a tedious task.

An egg salad or tuna salad sandwich also tastes excellent. Be very careful that the tuna salad does not contain MSG or MSG-containing flavoring, often hidden under various names. As I mentioned, many brands of tuna contain MSG; check the label before buying it.

Remember, if you are sensitive to MSG, any time you avoid buying MSG-containing food, you avoid eating it and spare yourself unpleasant symptoms. You also encourage the food manufacturer to prepare more food products without MSG. They want to make products you will buy.

Top off the sandwich with a pear or an apple to make the meal complete.

On the weekends I fix my own lunch. If I'm in a hurry, nothing beats a bagel, heated in a microwave, warm and smelling fragrantly of fresh-baked bread. It takes just a few more minutes to prepare a frozen chicken leg in the microwave. I dip into my supply of chicken legs, prepared by cooking a large number on the grill and basting them on one side with a very light coating of honey (even I cheat on the sugar avoidance at times). Alternatively, you can prepare chicken in the oven, dusted with a coating of crushed corn flakes.

In either preparation, when I worry about my fat intake (which I do far too infrequently), I remove the skin. After they cool, I wrap each leg in aluminum foil, freeze, and save for a future meal, when a quick trip to the microwave provides a nourishing entrée free of MSG.

I also enjoy another lunch, sausage—one without MSG in any of its names. As with the chicken, I precook the sausages, freeze them, and heat them before adding them to a delicious sandwich.

Or, if I have the time and the ambition, I will make a salad of lettuce, ripe olives, sliced onions, sunflower seeds, and perhaps sliced beef or turkey. I find this salad pleasing to the taste without salad dressing— skipping the salad dressing frees me from trying to find a salad dressing that does not contain sugar, MSG, tomatoes, or vinegar. (Olive oil sometimes seems right; vinegar is a product of fermentation and probably contains a small amount of fermentation-derived MSG. If you use a vinegar-based dressing, use grain-derived or white vinegar to avoid those made from wine or cider, with their attendant tartaric and citric acid.)

An egg salad or a tuna salad prepared with mayonnaise that doesn't contain citrus fruit juice or MSG can make a delightful lunch; add onions, celery, and any other ingredients that appeal to your palate. Remember to watch out for MSG in the tuna.

Dinner

The evening meal is a special meal—a time to relax after the hurry and bustle of the day. A time to reacquaint yourself with your family and to share experiences. A time to prepare for the events of the evening, whether these include a social engagement, a task that could not be completed during the day, or a quiet time with a good book.

Preparing a meal at home allows you to control its content, something that cannot be done when eating at a restaurant or a friend's home. I suspect this safe preparation encourages my patients to eat at home once they understand which foods and beverages they must avoid. Besides, they take great pride and satisfaction in preparing a delicious home-cooked meal.

One of my favorite dinners features fresh fish of any type, although my palate finds salmon the king of taste. Nesting the salmon on a bed of rice, especially wild rice, makes a delectable meal that I thoroughly enjoy.

If I'm in the mood for beef, a hamburger with lettuce, onions, and sliced pickles satisfies this craving. A nice salad, prepared as described previously, complements the meal.

If I want a more substantial piece of beef, I might choose a steak (such as my favorite, T-bone) broiled in the oven or barbecued on the grill, accompanied by asparagus (in season) or peas or beans, boiled well. Any of these meats mate well with corn sliced from the cob and boiled well.

I enjoy soups and stews for lunch or dinner. Although the soup you buy at the grocery often is often flavored with MSG-containing prepa-rations, the soup or stew you prepare at home shouldn't be. If you buy a soup or stew mix, just be careful it does not contain MSG. Look in the natural-foods section of your grocery, coop, or national marketers such as Whole Foods Market. The latter's Soup Bone 10 Bean Soup Mix looks just right.

In the mood for pork chops? Shake a few chops in a paper bag con-taining a mixture of flour and black pepper and fry them in a small amount of vegetable oil. The taste is outstanding.

Notice I have not included potatoes in my meals. For me, as for many of my patients, potatoes are too easily eaten in excess. Food-chemical-sensitive patients must limit how much potato they eat or they will experience the same symptoms caused by tomatoes. Many find that one or two servings of potatoes per week present no problem, but more than that causes discomfort. If patients are unsure of how much is too much, they had best not eat potatoes at all. For those more adventurous than I, enjoy your potatoes but limit the amount prudently.

Dessert

A sweet treat rewards you after a busy and productive day; it gives you a satisfying way to end the evening meal. Visions of cherry or lemon meringue pie or any of the exquisite-tasting ice creams, especially those with chocolate, must dance through the dreams of the unfortunate vic-tim of food allergy. I know they dance through the dreams of this victim.

Although I can't enjoy these fine desserts—my body complains loudly for days if I eat them—I have many fond childhood memories of finishing the evening meal with a delicious bowl of ice cream. Now I know that I can't eat that ice cream—I must avoid refined sugar. Many of my patients share my sensitivity.

For us, sweet foods and drinks are out. In addition, carbonated bev-erages with low-calorie sweeteners cannot replace beverages contain-ing refined sugar, nor can a dessert of delectable cheesecake (MSG) substitute for a slice of sugar-laden pie or cake.

To summarize the role of desserts in our diet: they belong in my patients' dreams and not in their stomachs. The same may be true for you. Unless someone comes up with a dessert that doesn't contain refined sugar, MSG, low-calorie sweeteners, or citrus-type acids, we food-sensitive people must be content with an apple, a pear, a banana, a peach, or a slice of melon. Although from these fruits emanate no aroma or flavor like a piping-hot slice of pie nor the smooth creamy texture of a dish of ice cream, they provide us with a healthy and safe alternative.

Snacks

Human nature rebels against a rigid schedule of three meals a day. A good example is our digestive system. Although we struggle to adapt it to regular meals, it refuses to respond to our struggle. It's like a baby awakening from a nap crying in hunger. Well before the next meal, our stomachs cry to be fed. We react to this demanding stomach by hunting for a snack.

Food manufacturers try to satisfy this between-meals demand. They make a large assortment of products that we can eat for snacks, and many taste great.

Which of these foods and beverages fit on our food allergy diet? You can answer this question by imagining yourself rummaging through the kitchen shelves and the refrigerator in search of a between-meals treat. You say to yourself, "My, that ice cream in the freezer looks good. On the other hand, those potato chips with that tasty cheese dip—how perfect for a snack. Or shall I choose the flavored corn chips, or those chocolate chip cookies? Maybe I should stick to my weight-loss diet, peel that juicy orange, and limit the pounds."

Of course, you decide to top off your snack delightfully with a high-citrus, high-sugar carbonated beverage. Aren't you glad you can find such delicious foods and beverages to please your tummy and satisfy your between-meals hunger and thirst?

Do not feel too glad. The snacks I just mentioned contain lots of refined sugar, MSG, citric and other acids, or low-calorie sweeteners.

I do not want to rob you of the satisfaction these snacks provide, but I do want to rob these food chemicals of their ability to cause your headaches, stomach aches, stuffiness, fuzzy thinking, and many other ailments. If you are food-chemical-sensitive, I want you to trade good taste for good health.

What Drinks and Snacks Can Food-Chemical-Sensitive People Eat and Drink?

Let's examine some snacks for the food-sensitive person so he or she knows how to satisfy that between-meals hunger. If you do not tolerate one or more of the foods or beverages I mention, don't eat them.

Beverages

Although alternatives exist for the prohibited snack *foods*, few alternatives exist for the *beverages* we enjoy and even crave. These beverages include those sweetened by refined sugar or low-calorie sweetener, whether carbonated or noncarbonated. My patients enjoy the taste of these beverages, but they do not enjoy the distress they cause. To avoid this distress, my patients must choose coffee, tea, water, or milk. In addition, like everyone else, they must avoid the excess caffeine of too much coffee and tea.

Those who must avoid sweetened and fruity beverages will find it handy (and a partial substitute for the sodas we all enjoy) to pour and drink a glass of carbonated mineral water, plain and not flavored. It somewhat quiets the desire for a beverage with citrus and sugar, a desire whose fulfillment they would later regret.

Sometimes the eating urge they feel is really a thirst signal—the body is really asking for water and not for food. At times we misinterpret this request for water as a desire for snacks. To counter this mistake, some diets specify drinking large amounts of water each day. This is wise advice, so when seized by the desire to snack, first try satisfying the urge to eat by drinking a glass of water.

Light Snacks

Often our craving for between-meals foods arises more from a desire to chew something than from a desire to load our stomachs with high-calorie food. If water does not satisfy the snack attack, consider celery and carrots—their crunchy taste may satisfy the desire to chew while at the same time supplying nourishment, vitamins, and minerals without a heavy calorie load.

Apples, bananas, peaches, and pears may also satisfy between-meals hunger. Most of our patients eat these nutritious fruits without provoking allergy symptoms. Another handy way to snack is to keep a container of cantaloupe, honeydew, or watermelon pieces stored in the refrigerator. A dishful of these red, yellow, or green fruits is as delightful to the taste buds as to the eyes.

Heavier Snacks

If a light snack will not satisfy the between-meals hunger pangs, here's where all the various breads come in handy. If they are free of raisins and free of or low in sugar, you can eat them freely. If you tolerate peanut butter, spread some on a slice of bread, but first read the label to be sure it is low in sugar and free of other problem ingredients.

Sometimes a slice of acceptable sandwich meat will strike your fancy, perhaps with a glass of milk. Or you might microwave some MSG-free breakfast sausage you have already precooked and stored in the freezer. A small piece of that chicken you cooked and froze may be just the right thing to appeal to your snack-hungry palate.

As you search for foods to tide you over until the next meal, don't forget the many varieties of crackers. Look for the ones free of MSG flavorings. Hopefully you purchased a brand low in or free of sugar, such as Nabisco Triscuits (the wheat and bran variety looks good to me) or Kavli Norwegian crispbread, an all-natural cracker made with whole-grain wheat, rye, water, and salt. Don't top them with cheese— eat them plain or with butter, margarine, or peanut butter.

Every time I think of crackers, I think of the number of brands with sugar listed second or third on the label. Crackers are not the only foods with sugar; many other foods also contain sugar. This worries me. If my patients eat enough of these foods, they will accumulate significant amounts of refined sugar.

That's why I hesitate to mention the sugared crackers here. An exception may be Sunshine Krispy Original Saltine Crackers, which lists sugar far down on the list of ingredients, which I hope means the quantity is small.

Although the snacks we discussed will satisfy your hunger, sometimes you would rather enjoy a crunchy chip snack. Regretfully, if you are sensitive to the food chemicals we are discussing, potato chips are not for you. But how about a plain corn chip, such as Old Dutch Restaurante Style Tortilla Chips or Deli Tostados? Or Frito-Lay Sun Chips, Original Flavor, with corn and other grains? (Sugar is listed sixth on the label.)

Although many of my patients suffer discomfort from corn, they may tolerate the corn in these chips. For those who need to go easy on fat, why not try the low-salt pretzels?

Any chip with flavoring added may, and often does, contain MSG, designated by the name monosodium glutamate or any other name including various "flavorings." Watch for this ingredient.

Shopping for Snacks

Do not hesitate to explore stores looking for snacks you can eat. To show you how a search can yield acceptable products, I wandered into our local Whole Foods Market to find snacks that might be acceptable to food-chemical-sensitive people. Many suitable foods lined the shelves.

I spied many varieties of potato chips without MSG flavoring, acceptable for those who can tolerate potato chips. I passed them up, as I tolerate potato chips poorly. I do, however, tolerate corn chips and found many varieties acceptable to our diet. One intrigued me: Red Chips by Garden of Eatin', Inc., grown from red corn; I purchased it. Another excellent alternative is Terra Sliced Sweet Potato Chips (made from yams and not Irish or white potatoes).

How about Instant Black Beans by Fantastic Foods? Just reconstitute by adding boiling water, and use as a chip dip.

I like smoked oysters, and so I purchased Smoked Oysters in Pure Olive Oil by Crown Prince. I also purchased Norda brand Zarte Herings-Filets in Senf-Dill-Creme, a product of Germany.

Pumpkin seeds called Roasted and Salted Pepitas by Bergin Nut Company, roasted in vegetable oil and salt, caught my eye and later proved delicious. Their Soy Nuts also looked like an interesting snack, and I bought and enjoyed them.

My purpose in listing these products is not necessarily to urge you to buy them but rather to illustrate the many varieties of snacks that should be acceptable to the food-chemical-sensitive person. I enjoy these snacks; you may like other snacks that I have not mentioned.

Seek out natural-food stores and coops, and look in the natural-foods section of your grocery store. They have selections of snacks that you should be able to tolerate that do not contain MSG, low-calorie sweeteners, excess refined sugar, or excess acid. These selections should fit any budget.

Two last snack suggestions: Number one: At a party seek out the shrimp—unless, of course, you are allergic to it—and enjoy it without the dip. I do. Number two: If you are spending the evening by yourself, pour a small amount of sunflower seeds (free of MSG flavoring) into a bowl, maybe add soy nuts, and prop your feet up in front of the TV. Enjoy the tube while you savor the sunflower seeds'/soy nuts' delicious, crunchy taste.

Dining Out

Even we who suffer from food allergy can eat at restaurants, enjoying the meal, smiling and laughing in the pleasant companionship of our fellow diners. We can leave the restaurant happy in the memories of sharing a satisfying meal with good friends, feeling as healthy as those who suffer no food allergy. To do this, we need to understand our food allergy and choose only the foods and beverages that we tolerate.

I remember a patient I treated many years ago. She endured her share of everyday worries. She did not seek out the extra troubles brought on by her diet. Unfortunately, her diet made her very uncomfortable, and my ineffective attempt to treat her forced my attention onto food allergy. At that time I did not know enough about foods to tell her how to dine without regret.

When we met, I found Marlene to be a pleasant young woman, the mother of three small children. Like so many of my patients, she suffered from a number of allergic illnesses, and hers included headaches, intermittent hives, and spring and fall hay fever. One symptom overshadowed the others, and it embarrassed her enormously. As she told me about it, our conversation went something like this.

"Marlene, do you have any trouble with food allergy?" I asked, as I reviewed the various illnesses that brought her to see me.

"Yes, I do have problems with foods, especially when I eat at a restaurant," she answered with a look on her face that convinced me she was reluctant to tell me about it.

"What's the problem, Marlene?"

"It's so embarrassing, Dr. Walsh," she said with a frown. "Having three little children, my husband and I seldom go out to eat, so when we do, it's really a major event, and we look forward to the evening with great anticipation. We usually invite good friends and combine dinner with a show.

"But we have to go to dinner an hour early because, after I eat, I have to spend an hour in the rest room with terrible diarrhea. I'm embarrassed, my husband is embarrassed, and I'm sure our friends think I'm peculiar."

I understood why Marlene was reluctant to tell me her story—her embarrassment made it difficult for her to discuss these traumatic events, even with me. I suspect she worried that I, too, would think she was peculiar. But I didn't. I saw how this food reaction placed a strain on her marriage and interfered cruelly with her limited social time. For her it was devastating.

At that time, although I sympathized with her, I couldn't help her because my limited knowledge of food allergy blinded me to the foods causing her embarrassment. In retrospect, after treating so many patients with similar diarrheas, I know that the foods causing her diarrhea were those carrying the chemicals that my food-sensitive patients must avoid.

Avoiding the Foods and Beverages That Cause Illness

When my patients or I eat in a restaurant, we must pay attention to the foods and beverages that turn the happy enjoyment of an excellent meal into unhappy pain and discomfort. Some of these foods and beverages we recognize easily; however, because we like them, we do not find them easy to avoid. (We need real willpower to progress from recognition to avoidance.) We find other foods hard to avoid, not so much because we like them but because we do not even know that their contents may trouble us.

The foods and beverages we find hard to recognize we will discuss later; for now, let's quickly review those that we recognize easily.

Refined sugar. If it tastes sweet, it is sweet, and probably loaded with refined sugar. Examples such as sweet rolls, sweet sauces, coffee with sugar, syrup, sweet carbonated beverages, pies, cakes, ice cream, cookies, and other treats spring quickly to mind. Food-sensitive patients should not eat or drink more of these foods and beverages than they can tolerate.

Low-calorie sweeteners. We meet these chemicals in low-calorie carbonated beverages and those little packets for sweetening coffee or tea. Pass them by.

Citrus. You should recognize foods and beverages containing high levels of citrus as easily as you recognize those loaded with refined sugar—as sugar tastes sweet, citrus and its sister acids taste fruity. Therefore, both citrus and sugar flavors are as easily identifiable as they are exceedingly delicious.

In the restaurant, we find citrus in breakfast juice, in fruit plates that include oranges or grapefruit, and in foods and beverages flavored with lime or lemon juice. Many sauces and salad dressings contain citrus— orange, tomato, berry; ask your server about the ingredients of the sauce or salad dressing before ordering it. Try cultivating a taste for salad without dressing.

We find citrus in the jelly or jamlike spreads used on bread. In addition, expect to find it in the many desserts, candies, and carbonated and noncarbonated beverages with a delectable fruity flavor—here it usually accompanies refined sugar. Either refuse these appealing treats or pass them on to a companion who can eat and drink them without pain and discomfort. (Sneaking a taste is okay.)

Harder to Recognize—Monosodium Glutamate (MSG)

MSG hides under many disguises in a restaurant meal, and three factors aid its concealment: (1) it is generally recognized as safe; (2) the chef can add it in many forms; and (3) many foods contain it in high levels naturally.

It is generally recognized as safe. Every cook worth his or her salary wants to prepare an excellent meal for the restaurant's patrons. One method of assuring delectable flavor in a meal is to add the flavoring agents and seasonings that contain MSG. (There is no question in my mind that MSG is a superlative flavoring agent; usually I can detect its presence in a meal because of the excellent flavor of the food I am eating.) Expect to find it in any meat or fish preparation. Expect it in soups, where its flavor brings a taste of extra robustness. Croutons also often contain it for the same reason.

The chef who adds MSG to a meal harbors no malicious desire to harm his or her patrons. The opposite is true. The chef would never use an additive in the meal if he or she even suspected that it caused harm. Moreover, there is no reason to suspect MSG; it sits proudly on the FDA's list of the safest food ingredients, the "generally recognized as safe (GRAS)" list.

Therefore, because the chef might not regard MSG as capable of causing his or her patrons distressing symptoms, he or she probably will not take pains to clearly indicate its presence in the food he or she prepares. The chef's patrons must realize that they need to ask about MSG to be sure that the food they eat does not contain this flavoring agent.

The chef can add it in many forms. Many seasonings and flavorings contain MSG, and unless a chef is especially knowledgeable about the contents of the flavorings and seasonings he or she uses, the chef may be using one of these flavorings without knowing it contains MSG. This is not surprising. The MSG content is high in seasonings containing the following ingredients: monosodium glutamate, MSG, hydrolyzed vegetable protein, autolyzed yeast extract, yeast extract, sodium and calcium caseinate, and even cheese and various forms of natural flavorings or natural flavor. With each of these products, the chef delivers significant quantities of MSG to the patron's meal. I often wonder if the chef who prepares my meal knows how much MSG it contains.

I admit I compound this uncertainty—I am not the brave type who calls for the chef and asks about the MSG content of the food. Instead, I ask the server, who then asks the chef. This chain of questions and answers allows more chance for confusion, especially as the server may not know anything about that strange chemical called MSG and may forget the name before he or she talks to the chef.

Many foods contain it in high levels naturally. Avoiding MSG in a restaurant meal is more complicated than just asking the server if the chef uses it in meal preparation. As discussed before, we encounter MSG in many natural, unmanufactured, or unprocessed foods. Unless you remember this and avoid these foods, you may eat a meal with too much MSG.

Tomatoes not only contain citrus, they also contain MSG. Tomato sauces concentrate this MSG and acid. Corn also contains it, but corn separated from the cob and then boiled until soft may contain less. Mushrooms have it, as do many preparations made with seaweed or kelp (forms of algae). Any fermented or aged food contains MSG— well-aged cheese has surprisingly high levels of MSG, as does soy sauce. My patients must be careful that their restaurant meal does not contain these foods and flavorings.

Choosing a Meal at a Restaurant

We have looked at the restaurant foods and beverages with problem ingredients. Now let's try to answer the question my patients ask when they go to a restaurant. What can they eat?

The answer for them and for you: Select your meal carefully, and don't feel alone. Many other people and I must carefully scrutinize the menu because we also suffer the untoward effects of these chemicals. Perhaps some of the avoidance methods I practice may help you order wisely so that you feel well after the meal.

Breakfast. For me, breakfast is easy to order. I often order pancakes and an egg, sunny side up. Because of its sugar content, I do not use syrup, but I like to top the pancakes with something, so I place the egg on top of the pancakes and add salt and pepper. This combination satisfies me.

Another breakfast I order is oatmeal or Cream of Wheat, perhaps with a side order of well-cooked bacon and a banana or a slice of melon—no sausage, as it may be flavored with MSG. Some of the dry breakfast cereals, low in refined sugar, also would be acceptable.

Sometimes the restaurant serves breakfast buffet-style, where I can choose from a large selection of breakfast foods. If I find fish selections, cooked without sauce or breading (which may contain MSG), I load my plate. I enjoy fish. Next, I look for the fruit section and slowly, one by one, load my plate with watermelon and other melon slices while dodging strawberries and pineapples. I skip the juice and use water or skim milk for my beverage. For the meat course I choose bacon or other sliced meats—free of sauce and breading that may contain MSG.

Someday I hope I will be able to choose breaded foods or foods prepared in sauce. I was encouraged that this day may not be far off when I talked to one of my patients who is chief of catering at a large and famous hotel in St. Paul—she tells me her catering service does not use MSG in seasoning their meals.

Although I believe that many food preparers no longer use MSG because of concern about its effect on diners, I still avoid sauces and breading that may contain it. I don't know which preparers still use this seasoning under its own name or any of the many other sanitized names that hide the MSG content.

The day may come when, as we puzzle over which dishes to choose, we see a little sign telling us which selections do not contain MSG under any name and which do—and the amount present. That sign I would find most helpful, and it would be most deeply appreciated.

Lunch and dinner. I find the problems of food selection in a restaurant similar whether I am ordering lunch or dinner, so let's examine the noon and evening meals together.

At both meals, as I peruse the menu, I look for main courses that are simply prepared. I immediately eliminate from consideration all meat, poultry, and fish prepared in sauces or marinated and choose a simply processed slice of meat such as a steak, asking the server to make sure the chef adds no seasoning. By asking for no seasoning instead of asking for no MSG, I believe I avoid the need to teach the server about MSG and all the seasonings preparations in which it may be found. Add your own salt and pepper.

No seasoning means no MSG, and this simple instruction also means no confused server trying to tell the chef not to add that strange seasoning, the name of which may be forgotten on the way to the kitchen.

Don't assume that because a restaurant is expensive, it does not use MSG to season its steaks. I have made this mistake. I have ordered food in excellent, expensive restaurants where I assumed the steak was so good the chef would not add seasoning. I found that naive thought was wrong. The chef added MSG to all meat dishes without warning patrons by noting its use in the menu.

On two occasions I discovered this after the server brought the steak; sheepishly, I had to send it back. I felt like a fool because I forgot to ask about MSG when I ordered the meal, but each time, in spite of this guilty feeling, I still sent back the steak. Of course I apologized, but I was also irritated. Why do they add MSG and not tell the patron? Because the chef does not realize it causes people like me pain and discomfort.

At one of the restaurants of a national chain I discovered that my cautious use of the no-seasoning order did me no good. When I detected the taste of MSG in my steak, I asked the waitress why it was used in spite of my instructions. She asked the cook and relayed the answer to me. The cook had not seasoned my food. All the food comes to the restaurant preseasoned with MSG. I now ask if the food is pre-seasoned before ordering.

If I order fish, I make sure it is prepared without sauces and seasonings. An herb-butter preparation is fine, as are almonds, and both impart a great flavor to the fish.

Salads are a problem. I have learned to eat salad without dressing, and I even find it enjoyable (it took me three years to get used to the taste). Because vinegar is a fermented product, it may contain some quantity of MSG. However, if the food-allergic diner finds a salad without dressing distasteful, try olive oil by itself or vinegar and oil; they probably are the safest. Be sure the vinegar is white vinegar made from grains and not any of the vinegars made from wine or cider, which contain citric and tartaric acids.

Avoid all salad dressings with tomatoes, cheese, citrus juices, and sugar. Unfortunately, that includes almost all dressings other than oil and vinegar.

At a buffet-type lunch or dinner, follow the advice we discussed for a cafeteria-style breakfast. Confine your fruit to apples, pears, bananas, melons, and peaches. Lettuce, carrots, celery, onions, ripe olives, beans, sunflower seeds, eggs, and coleslaw are acceptable for a salad. In any pasta salad, examine the dressing for a crumbly appearance—it probably signifies aged cheese that has been added to enhance the flavor. As we discussed, aged cheese is naturally high in MSG because fermentation breaks the milk protein of the cheese into its component amino acids, releasing MSG.

If you must have a dish prepared in a sauce, ask the waiter, waitress, or chef if it contains wine or MSG, or any seasoning with MSG (and hope whoever you ask knows the many different names of the seasonings that contain MSG). To be safe, and if the choice is available, select meat or fish that is sliced by the chef while you wait. Your chance of eating preseasoned food will be less.

What if you are invited to a restaurant meal where the menu is set and you cannot choose your own food? Do what I do: eat beforehand.

Then, if the food contains the dietary chemicals I must avoid, I eat only the safe part of the meal and tell anyone who notices that I am not hungry. It's the truth—because of my prior meal. (Eating beforehand prevents my stomach from overruling my head.)

In Defense of the Restaurant Staff

In my previous remarks, I made the assumption that the restaurant staff possess little knowledge of MSG and its allergic effects. This assumption was valid in the past, but it is becoming less true with time.

My recent experiences show me that, at least in the restaurants I frequent, both the cooking and serving staff know about MSG and help you avoid it when you ask. To these knowledgeable people, sorry about the unkind remarks.

However, if the chef uses an MSG-containing flavoring not clearly labeled as containing MSG, servers may not know that it is in the food they recommend. In addition, they probably do not know that a preparation with soy sauce, mushrooms, tomatoes, or aged cheese contains lots of MSG. So, when asking your servers for advice on your selections, be sure you use your own knowledge to supplement theirs.

Food allergy patients can enjoy a meal in a restaurant. Yes, their choices are limited. Yes, they have to abstain from some of the most delicious selections on the menu. But when the meal is finished, they won't suffer food allergy's painful symptoms. They will avoid its headaches and cramping abdominal pains. Their skin will not itch, their noses will not block, they will not see their bathroom scales groan under the bloated water weight, and their thinking will not be slowed by the foods they ate. They will relish the wonderful feeling that comes from eating properly.

Recipes for the Food Allergy Diet

As a diplomate of the American Board of Allergy and Immunology, I am trained in the treatment of patients with food allergy. However, being a specialist in treating food-sensitive patients does not mean I am a specialist in the food sciences.

I can diagnose food allergy and instruct my patients to avoid offending foods. However, my specialty training has not prepared me to prescribe a diet with the knowledge and authority of a registered dietician. They have the qualifications necessary to ensure meeting nutritional needs while formulating meal plans and menus for people whose health requires a special diet.

Recognizing this limitation, I was delighted when Felicia Busch agreed to put her specialty to work helping my patients. Felicia brings many unique qualifications to this task, not the least of which is that she is a registered member and charter fellow of the American Dietetic Association.

She is an experienced radio and TV guest expert in nutrition and an author. Among her works are *The New Nutrition: From Antioxidants to Zucchini* and many chapters for Mayo Clinic books on health and nutrition.

On the following pages Felicia provides information on nutrition, shopping tips, menu plans, and recipes to increase our patients' success with using the diet.

WHAT'S LEFT TO EAT?
by Felicia Busch, M.P.H., R.D.

What's left to eat? I have been asked that question at least a thousand times by patients who have had to make changes in their diets for a variety of reasons. Whether it's food allergy restrictions, a low-cholesterol diet, or a low-sodium diet, the first reaction is to think that there is nothing worth eating left on your list. Try, instead, to focus on all the wonderful foods you have to choose from.

Right now it's most important to concentrate on the changes in your diet needed to make you feel better. The following dietary guidelines for Americans are the bases of sound eating for healthy adults. Use these guidelines as a model for planning your food choices, but keep in mind that eliminating foods that cause you harm is your main priority now. A balanced diet is something to achieve over time, not overnight.

The Dietary Guidelines for Americans

Eat a variety of foods to get the energy, proteins, vitamins, minerals, and fiber you need for good health.

Maintain a healthy weight to reduce your chances of having high blood pressure, heart disease, certain cancers, and diabetes. Choose a diet low in fat, saturated fat, and cholesterol to reduce your risk of heart disease and certain types of cancer. Because fat contains more than twice the calories of other foods, a diet low in fat can help you maintain a healthy weight.

Choose a diet with plenty of vegetables, fruits, and grain products, which provide needed vitamins, minerals, fiber, and complex carbohydrates.

Use sugars only in moderation. A diet with lots of sugars has too many calories and too few nutrients for most people and can help cause tooth decay.

Use salt and sodium only in moderation to help reduce your risk of high blood pressure.

If you drink alcoholic beverages, do so in moderation. Alcoholic beverages supply calories but little or no nutritional value.

Following Through

It has been my experience in more than fifteen years as a registered dietician that people with food allergies are more likely to be faithful to their special diets. You will actually feel much better when you eliminate problem foods. And there is nothing like feeling great to help reinforce the benefits of a new way of eating. After the initial anxiety of eliminating or reducing many of your favorite foods, you'll find there are lots of delicious and nutritious foods you can eat that will make you feel good.

It does take extra time and planning to follow any special diet. Budget more time at the grocery store to read food labels. You'll need extra minutes in the kitchen to make some recipes from scratch. Try to keep your kitchen stocked with staples. In that way, at the end of a busy day you won't have to worry about what to fix for dinner—you'll have all the basic ingredients on hand.

I find it helpful to sketch out menus a week in advance. You don't have to plan down to the last detail, but a rough idea will help you stay on track. To help you get started, I have put together a week's worth of sample menus and recipes that fit the specific requirements of Dr. Walsh's dietary recommendations. Remember that one diet will not work for everyone; each individual has his or her own specific nutrient needs and reactions to foods. Adapt these suggestions to meet your particular needs, adding or subtracting foods as necessary. *Bon appétit!*

Tips for High-Nutrition Shopping

Any type of dietary limitation requires careful attention to be sure that a wide enough variety of foods is included to guarantee a balanced diet. To choose foods rich in vitamins and minerals, consider the following recommendations:

When buying breads, grains, rice, and pasta: Choose whole-grain varieties whenever possible; they contain more B vitamins and fiber than refined products. Read the label of breads to see if whole-grain flour is listed first.

Choose cooked and ready-to-eat cereals with no more than two grams of fat and at least two grams of fiber per serving. Avoid cereals with added sugar.

When buying fruits and vegetables: Choose loose leaf lettuce such as romaine and endive, which contain many nutrients, instead of iceberg lettuce, with few nutrients. Choose dark green broccoli and deep orange carrots instead of poorly colored ones. Darkly colored green and yellow vegetables have more vitamins and minerals than lightly colored ones.

Choose fresh fruits and vegetables in season to provide maximum nutrition. When foods are not in season or look inferior in quality, choose plain frozen varieties.

Purchase canned fruits packed in water or juice, and drain before using. Eat at least five servings of fruits and vegetables a day for good health.

When buying dairy products: Choose low-fat and skim milk foods instead of whole milk varieties. Limit your intake of cheese, and choose only plain yogurt. The fermentation process used to manufacture such products releases MSG. Some individuals may not tolerate any cheese or yogurt; others can eat limited amounts.

When buying meat, poultry, and seafood: Choose lean, well-trimmed, fresh cuts of meat whenever possible. Remove all skin and fat from poultry before cooking. Choose lean ground beef and drain all excess fat while cooking. Choose fresh or frozen fish and seafood without breading, tuna packed in water. Check canned tuna for added MSG. Always read the label of processed meats to see if MSG or MSG-containing flavorings are added. Product formulations change frequently, so read and check labels each time you buy.

Foods to Keep on Hand

Breads, Grain, Rice, and Cereals

(six to eleven servings recommended per day)

Plain white, whole-wheat, and other whole-grain breads
Bagels and English muffins
White and whole-wheat flour
White and whole-wheat flour tortillas
White, brown, and wild rice
Pasta and noodles, assorted shapes and sizes
Oatmeal
Cold cereals (without added sugar)
Hot cereals

Vegetables

(three to five servings recommended per day)

Artichokes
Asparagus
Beets
Broccoli, boiled only
Cabbage, boiled only
Carrots
Celery
Corn, cut off the cob
   and boiled only
Cucumbers
Green beans
Lettuce
Okra
Olives, without pimento
Onion
Parsnips
Radishes
Rutabagas
Squash
Yams, sweet potatoes

Fruits

(two to four servings recommended per day)

Apples
Bananas
Cantaloupe
Honeydew melon

Peaches
Pears
Nectarines
Watermelon

Dairy Products

(two to three servings recommended per day)

Milk (skim, low-fat, or whole)

Meats and Meat Alternatives

(two servings recommended per day)

Beef
Chicken
Fresh pork

Tuna (avoid canned varieties
   with added MSG)
Turkey

Seasonings

Basil
Cinnamon
Garlic powder or salt
Nutmeg
Onion powder or salt
Oregano

Pepper
Salt
Vanilla
White vinegar (do not substitute
   flavored vinegars)

Suggested Menus

(an asterisk after an item indicates that its recipe is included in this section)

Day 1

BREAKFAST

Scrambled egg

Lean Canadian bacon

Toast with margarine

Cantaloupe slice

Coffee, tea, or milk

LUNCH

Grilled or baked chicken sandwich with lettuce

Carrot and celery sticks

Fresh apple

Milk

DINNER

Meatloaf

Green beans, boiled

Herbed white rice

Dinner roll with margarine

Milk

Day 2

BREAKFAST

Oatmeal

Bagel with margarine or butter

Coffee, tea, or milk

LUNCH

Spinach salad

Oil and white vinegar dressing*

Bacon bits and chopped egg, if desired

Whole-grain bread with margarine

Canned peaches and pear slices, packed in juice and drained before eating

Milk

DINNER

Pork chop

Cabbage, boiled well

Sweet potato

Rye bread with margarine

Milk

Day 3

BREAKFAST
Puffed cereal
Banana
Toast with margarine
Coffee, tea, or milk

LUNCH
Plain hamburger with lettuce,
    onion, pickles, and mustard
    (check mustard for MSG)
Side salad
Oil and white vinegar dressing*
Apple
Milk

DINNER
Broiled fish
Cooked carrots
Marinated cucumbers*
Dinner roll with margarine
Milk

Day 4

BREAKFAST
French toast
Mashed fruit for topping, made
    from allowed fruits
Coffee, tea, or milk

LUNCH
Burrito made with tortilla filled
    with ground beef, chopped
    lettuce, and onion
Watermelon chunks or allowable
    fruit in season
Milk

DINNER
Homemade chicken and
    noodles*
Beets
Tossed salad
Oil and white vinegar dressing*
Milk

Day 5

BREAKFAST

Shredded wheat

Milk

Honeydew melon

LUNCH

Salad Nicoise*

Fruit cup, peaches, pears, apple
   chunks (rinse if canned)

Milk

DINNER

Steak

Mashed rutabaga with
   margarine

Broccoli, boiled

Tossed salad

Oil and white vinegar dressing*

Milk

Day 6

BREAKFAST

Buttermilk pancakes*

Mashed fruit for topping (from
   allowed fruits)

Coffee, tea, or milk

LUNCH

Pasta Primavera*

Whole-grain bread with margarine

Milk

DINNER

Roast turkey with homemade
   gravy

Yams or squash

Green beans, boiled

Bread stuffing*

Baking powder biscuits with
   margarine

Milk

Day 7

BREAKFAST

Banana muffins*

Stewed apples

Coffee, tea, or milk

LUNCH

Roast beef sandwich with
    lettuce and sprouts

Fresh pear

Pretzels

Milk

DINNER

Oven-baked chicken

Seasoned wild rice*

Corn, cut off the cob and boiled

Dinner roll with margarine

Milk

Recipes

Note: Whenever you use sugar in a recipe, be sure to limit carefully the total amount of additional sugar consumed per day.

Main Dishes

HOMEMADE CHICKEN AND NOODLES

3- to 4-pound chicken

1 pound egg noodles

1 medium onion

1 cup celery, diced

2 tablespoons margarine or butter

¼ cup flour

1 teaspoon salt

⅛ teaspoon pepper

Paprika

Boil chicken in 6 cups water until tender, about 2½ hours. Reserve 4 cups chicken broth. Remove chicken from bones in large pieces. Prepare noodles according to package directions and drain. Sauté onion and celery in margarine or butter until tender; stir in flour and mix well. Combine chicken, noodles, reserved broth, onion, celery, salt, and pepper. Pour into two 2-quart casseroles or one very large casserole. Bake uncovered at 350° for 30 minutes. Sprinkle top with paprika. Freeze one casserole for later use if desired.

MEAT LOAF

1 pound ground beef

¼ cup bread crumbs

½ cup milk

1 egg, beaten

Salt and pepper to taste

Mix all ingredients thoroughly. Shape into loaf and bake at 350° for 1 hour.

PASTA PRIMAVERA

½ pound pasta, regular to thin style

2 cups broccoli, boiled

3 large carrots, sliced and cooked

1 cup corn, cut from cob and boiled

⅔ cup olive oil

¼ cup white vinegar (do not substitute flavored
  vinegar)

¼ cup parsley, chopped

2 tablespoons dried basil (use ¼ cup if fresh)

1 clove garlic

½ teaspoon salt

¼ teaspoon pepper

Cook pasta according to package directions. Rinse in cold water and drain well. In large bowl, combine broccoli, carrots, and corn. Add pasta and toss gently. In blender or food processor, blend oil, vinegar, parsley, basil, garlic, salt, and pepper until smooth. Pour over pasta and toss.

SALAD NICOISE

¾ cup olive oil

¼ cup white vinegar (do not substitute flavored
  vinegar)

2 tablespoons chopped parsley

Salt and pepper to taste

¼ pound whole green beans, cooked

4 cups mixed salad greens

3 hard-cooked eggs cut into wedges

6¾-ounce can tuna, drained (check label to be sure
  MSG is not added)

1 small onion, cut into rings

Combine oil, vinegar, parsley, salt, and pepper to make dressing. Toss 2 tablespoons over the green beans and marinate 30 minutes. Arrange salad greens on plate. Arrange green beans, eggs, tuna, and onion over greens. Top with dressing or serve on the side.

Side Dishes

BREAD STUFFING

¼ cup minced onion

½ cup butter or margarine

4½ cups soft bread cubes, not store-bought

2 stalks celery with leaves, chopped

1 teaspoon salt

1 teaspoon sage

½ teaspoon thyme

½ teaspoon black pepper

In large skillet, cook and stir onion in butter or margarine until tender. Stir in about a third of bread cubes. Pour bread and onion mixture into bowl and add remaining bread and spices. Mix well. Press into baking dish and bake at 350° for 45 minutes.

Sausage stuffing variation: Decrease bread cubes to 4 cups and omit salt. Add ½ pound crumbled cooked sausage. (Be sure to read entire ingredient list to ensure that no MSG has been added to the sausage.)

MARINATED CUCUMBERS

2–3 medium cucumbers

1 tablespoon salt

¾ cup white vinegar (do not substitute flavored
    vinegars)

1 tablespoon sugar

¼ teaspoon pepper

Wash cucumbers and pat dry. Cut into paper-thin slices. Place slices in deep bowl and sprinkle every few layers with the 1 tablespoon salt. Let stand at room temperature for 2 hours. Drain thoroughly. Stir together remaining ingredients and pour over slices. Cover and refrigerate at least 4 hours. Drain cucumbers before serving.

OIL AND WHITE VINEGAR DRESSING

⅔ cup salad oil

½ cup white vinegar (do not substitute flavored vinegar)

2 teaspoons dried mustard

1 teaspoon dried basil, crushed

1 teaspoon dried oregano, crushed

½ teaspoon dried dillweed

In screw-top jar, combine all ingredients and shake well to mix. Keep chilled in refrigerator and shake again before serving. Dressing tastes best if allowed to sit at least 24 hours before first use.

SEASONED WILD RICE

1 cup uncooked wild rice

½ cup margarine or butter

4 tablespoons chopped onion

2 stalks celery, chopped

½ teaspoon garlic salt

Wash and rinse dry rice. Place rice in heavy saucepan with 4 cups lightly salted water. Bring to a boil, then cover and simmer for 45 minutes. Uncover and fluff with a fork. Let stand an additional 5 to 10 minutes. Melt margarine or butter in saucepan and sauté onion and celery. Toss garlic salt, rice, and sautéed vegetables together to mix well.

Breakfast

BASIC MUFFIN BATTER

1 egg
1 cup milk
¼ cup salad oil
2 cups flour
¼ cup sugar
3 teaspoons baking powder
1 teaspoon salt

*The amount of sugar per muffin is just 1 teaspoon. You may choose to decrease the amount even further, but the muffins will lose some of their moistness and texture.

Heat oven to 400°. Grease the bottoms of 12 muffin cups or spray with cooking oil. Beat egg, and stir in milk and oil. Mix in remaining ingredients just until flour is moistened. Batter should be lumpy. Fill muffin cup two-thirds full. Bake for 20 to 25 minutes or until golden brown. Immediately remove from pan. Makes 12 muffins.

VARIETY MUFFINS

Apple: Stir in 1 cup grated apple and add ½ teaspoon cinnamon. Bake for 25 to 30 minutes.

Banana: Stir in 1 large or 2 small, very ripe, mashed bananas. Add 1 teaspoon vanilla. Bake for 25 to 30 minutes.

Oatmeal: Decrease white flour to one cup and add one cup oats.

Whole wheat: Decrease white flour to 1 cup and add 1 cup whole-wheat flour. Decrease baking powder to 2 teaspoons.

BUTTERMILK PANCAKES

2 cups sifted flour

1 teaspoon baking soda

1 teaspoon salt

1 tablespoon sugar*

2 eggs

2 cups buttermilk

2 tablespoons margarine, melted

*The amount of sugar per serving of pancakes is less than one teaspoon. You may choose to eliminate the sugar altogether.

Heat oiled griddle until hot. Sift together flour, soda, salt, and sugar. In separate bowl mix eggs, buttermilk, and margarine. Mix wet and dry ingredients together with spoon until just mixed. Batter will be lumpy. Spoon batter onto griddle and turn when top surface is full of bubbles. Turn only once.

CANTALOUPE COOLER

1 cup cantaloupe, cut into large chunks

½ cup milk, very cold

1 teaspoon vanilla

Whirl all ingredients in blender. Makes a refreshing 12-ounce drink.

CHAPTER 3

Integrating Our Knowledge of MALS and Classic Food Allergies

Contrasting MALS and Classic Food Allergy

We have explored allergy to food chemicals, also known as MALS food allergy. You will better understand food allergy if we now spend a little time examining how MALS food allergy and food-protein or classic food allergy compare. We will pay particular attention to:

◇ how they affect you
◇ the number of foods involved
◇ using blood and skin tests to diagnose food allergy
◇ how these food allergies cause your symptoms
◇ how health care professionals accept these food allergies

How They Affect You

Both types of food allergy can cause quick-acting symptoms; both also can set off delayed symptoms.

With either MALS or classic food allergy, a tiny amount of food may make you suffer a severe, even dangerous reaction. Or you may not react to a tiny amount of food; before symptoms start, you may need to eat an amount of food large enough to overpower your tolerance.

Therefore, both allergies can make your symptoms appear quickly while you eat, or hours after your meal while you relax, digesting your food.

The Number of Foods Involved

The proteins of foods tend to be specific for each food. For instance, shrimp protein is found in shrimp and not in milk. Similarly, milk protein is not found in chicken. (Okay, that's not always the case, but for now let's exclude proteins that are identical in different foods.)

Because classic food allergy is directed against the protein of foods, and because these proteins are specific to the food, classic food allergy tends to involve only one food or a limited number of foods. (Okay, that's not always the case either, as some patients react to many foods. But to make my point, let's exclude these patients.)

In contrast, MALS food allergy depends on the chemical content of the foods you eat, and a large number of foods contain excess quantities of these chemicals. Therefore, in contrast to classic food allergy sufferers, MALS sufferers typically react to a large number of foods. For instance, you find MSG in sausages, soups, and sandwiches; sugar in cookies, cakes, and candy; acid foods in oranges, cherries, berries, and beverages.

In summary, MALS food allergy tends to involve many foods; classic food allergy tends to involve one or a few.

Using Blood and Skin Tests to Diagnose Food Allergy

Blood tests measure allergy to proteins, classic food allergy. They measure quick-appearing food protein allergies (immediate classic food allergy) best, although at times they miss this diagnosis. They poorly measure or completely fail to measure delayed food protein allergy (delayed classic food allergy)

Therefore, for all practical purposes blood tests for foods measure only quick-reacting classic food allergy. They do not measure chemical allergy to foods; therefore, MALS food allergy cannot be diagnosed using blood tests.

Skin tests as currently performed measure only allergy to protein; again, only classic food allergy. If your primary caregiver or an allergist tests your skin for food allergy, the tests will attempt to measure allergy to food protein, not food chemicals. Like the blood tests, they measure best the quick-reacting classic food allergy. Using skin tests to diagnose delayed classic food allergy is possible but is seldom done.

Testing for the chemicals that cause MALS allergy is also seldom done. When performed, reactions to these chemicals are different from those that diagnose classic food allergy.

In this book I am trying to avoid discussing blood and skin tests. For a variety of reasons, many of you will have no opportunity to have either test performed. For example, your medical care professional may use another test to measure your allergy. Alternatively, your medical care professional may not test you because he or she is convinced that your symptoms are not caused by food allergy.

Do not overestimate the value of blood and skin tests. Although I find them valuable, they often frustrate me because they can miss food allergies that my patients find very important. Then we look for these allergies with elimination diets.

If you have skin tests performed, use their results to suggest foods to watch, and never accept them as gospel unless your dietary experiments confirm the tests. If you are denied the opportunity for tests, do not feel defeated. Using the concepts we discussed, you should still be able to identify troubling foods and find your own best diet.

How These Food Allergies Cause Your Symptoms

Getting hit by allergy is like being struck by a bullet. Allergy is not the bullet. It is not even the barrel, stock, or cylinder of the gun that shoots the bullet. The immune system makes up all these parts of the gun; it is responsible for the bullet that wounds you.

Food allergy, both MALS and classic, is only the finger that pulls the trigger. By itself, without the actions of the immune system, allergy causes no harm—it is as innocent as a baby with a powdered bottom and a full stomach, asleep in the crib. Unfortunately, although innocent, it still pulls the trigger.

When MALS and classic food allergy trigger the immune system they set off that system's attacking lymphocytes, illness-causing chemicals and hard-hitting antibodies that make your head hurt and your stomach ache.

As they both pull the same trigger—and launch the same immune system—these two food allergies cause the same symptoms. Their symptoms are often identical.

How Health Care Professionals Accept
These Food Allergies

As I mentioned, if you ask an allergist about food allergy, he or she will tell you about classic but probably not MALS food allergy. Of the points we discussed, the allergist may not agree to the following:

◇ that food allergy is common
◇ that patients can find their own food allergies
◇ that hidden immediate and delayed food allergy often exist and worsen other allergy symptoms such as hay fever
◇ that MALS food allergy exists
◇ that treating environmental allergy also treats food allergy

For instance, although I notice that many of my pollen-sensitive patients suffer less if they avoid allergic foods in the pollen seasons, other allergists believe that food allergy does not worsen pollen allergy. Similarly, although I find that calming environmental allergy also calms food allergy, other allergists do not think these allergies are related. This disagreement is only natural. We allergists treat a complicated illness that forces us to answer complicated questions. Are our patient's headaches, muscle aches, rashes, tiredness, or eating disorders caused by allergy? Which exposures in the home or at work cause trouble? Which foods make a patient miserable? What can be done to help a patient find release from suffering?

As allergists, we constantly struggle to answer these questions. As human beings, each with our own deeply held beliefs, our answers often differ.

To find an allergist who shares my approach to treating food allergy, call your local allergists and ask them if they test for and treat food allergy. Many will answer honestly that they do not assign a high priority to food allergy or that they diagnose and treat only immediate classic food allergy (food protein allergy).

I hope that you find an allergist knowledgeable in food allergy. If you do not, try to find another medical professional who can help you discover and treat your food allergies.

If you do not find an allergist who treats food allergy, you must treat yourself. I have written this book to assist you in this endeavor. I have tried to lead you gently from one concept to another, from one step in treatment to the next.

I have repeated some of these concepts, hoping that I could lock them in your mind. I hope that they are so locked in your mind that when your friend or a medical caregiver tells you foods cannot worsen your depression or make your hives flare, you will not be led astray; that if they tell you that foods cannot cause delayed reactions, you will not close your mind to this possibility.

Why do foods make us suffer? Formulating my answer to this question helped me to better understand food allergy. The answer should help you understand food allergy, and I will share this answer with you in the next section.

Why We Are Allergic to Foods

I know I share your desire to know why certain foods trouble us. When I began to realize the complexity of food allergy, it became apparent that my patients were reacting to a variety of foods, and that they would be forced to avoid a surprising number of foods and beverages, and I didn't have any idea why this was so. What made these seemingly different foods and beverages so troublesome? The foods and beverages are different—orange juice differs from diet soda, and cheese is not the same as soy sauce—but in many of my patients they cause the same symptoms as if they were the same foods and beverages. Orange juice, diet pop, cheese, and soy sauce all brought on the same headaches or hives or diarrhea.

I was learning how to treat my food-sensitive patients, but I was not learning why my treatment worked. I was irritated and frustrated.

The Usual Explanation of Food Allergy: Classic Food Allergy

One explanation of food allergy is widely accepted by allergists, and it explains how classic or food-protein allergy happens. Let's see if we can follow it.

All animal- and vegetable-derived foods are made up of proteins in addition to fats and carbohydrates. Many of the food proteins are identical to our own body's protein, and even allergic people absorb and digest them with no difficulty. But some food proteins are not like our body proteins. They are found in such foods as shrimp or nuts or cow's milk but not in our own bodies, and our bodies do not recognize them. In the allergic person, these unfamiliar or strange proteins lead to trouble.

When these strange shrimp, nut, or milk proteins gain entrance into the bloodstream, they are seized by the immune system, which starts the immune reaction, bringing on allergy symptoms. If an antibody called IgE is involved with the immune response, the body reacts alarmingly. Even tiny amounts of these foods make IgE release chemicals that welt the skin in hives, partially obstructing the small air passages in the lungs, causing wheezing, and partially blocking the large air passages, causing choking. The chemicals also dilate the blood vessels, dropping the blood pressure and threatening shock and unconsciousness.

This is an irrational overreaction by a body's system to a harmless food protein, much like shooting a mosquito off your leg with a shotgun. Unfortunately, for weeks, months, or a lifetime, the allergic person who reacts quickly to foods is stuck with it.

If lymphocytes or other antibodies—such as the IgG and IgM antibodies—react with this foreign food in the bloodstream, symptoms are considerably delayed. Then arise the chronic and persistent flulike symptoms of delayed classic food allergy. In contrast to the IgE antibody reaction, tiny amounts do not set off symptoms, only excess amounts—overloads.

Why does this reaction to food exist? It exists because we live in a sea of germs—viruses and bacteria that assault us from the air, water, and ground. Battling these pestilent germs, our immune systems act like vigilant bodyguards, striking so quickly that they destroy the germs before the germs kill us. Literally, our survival depends on their protection. If they failed, germs would mount devastating infections, killing us within hours.

Unfortunately, this protection creates a problem. As our immune systems hunt for the germs that would kill us, they sometimes fail to distinguish between what is harmful and what is devoid of harm. They attack harmless dust, mold, pollen, substances from pets, and food—which carry no threat of harm—as viciously as they attack germs. When they attack these harmless allergens, they create allergy.

This senseless attack on harmless molds, pollens, foods, and other allergens causes all the painful and uncomfortable symptoms that affect allergic people. It's why we sneeze and wheeze, why our skin itches and our noses stuff up. It brings on all the other symptoms we call allergies.

Although we resent suffering these symptoms, we must not blame our immune systems. Instead, remember that they keep us alive in a germ-filled world. They do not mean to hurt us; our pain and discomfort are only undesirable side effects of their vital protection.

Controlling the Immune System

All of us, whether or not we suffer allergies, possess this protective immune bodyguard. We are all allergic to foods.

To counteract this allergy, we also have traffic cops roaming our bloodstream. As soon as they notice our immune system attacking harmless food, they throw up roadblocks. They stop the immune system before it makes our head hurt or our skin itch.

If everybody shares allergies to foods and everybody has a police force to stop these reactions, why do some of us suffer from food allergy? Because, in food allergy sufferers, the police force is weak. It fails to stop food allergy reactions.

This does not have to be a lifelong failure. Earlier in life many of us suffered no allergic symptoms; our police seemed adequate. For months or years, they prevented food allergy symptoms and we lived free from this distressing problem. However, eventually their weakness showed. Too few of them guard against food reactions, and those that do guard weaken with age. They move too slowly to stop the frantically rushing immune system.

For some people the weakness involves only one or a few foods. Perhaps the control for shrimp or strawberries just isn't up to its task. For others, the weakness extends through all the foods in the diet, and they react to all foods, some foods bringing more symptoms than other foods.

Why We React to Food Chemicals—MALS Food Allergy

The reason for MALS food allergy is different. I don't know if the following explanation is correct, but I think it is; I know it helps me understand why my patients suffer from MALS food allergy.

To understand the explanation, it helps to compare your body's cells to miniature cities. They are special cities, not at all like our present-day metropolises, which use electricity, oil, and natural gas for power. Instead, the cell cities in our bodies use a miracle fuel as powerful as nuclear fuel but without many of its dangers.

This marvelous fuel has to be handled carefully. Instead of being shoveled or pumped into a furnace, to be consumed by fire all at once, it goes through a series of furnaces, each furnace releasing energy to the cell by burning only part of the fuel. When the last furnace finishes, a special chemical renews the spent fuel and the whole cycle of energy production starts again. A complicated process to produce power, but tremendously efficient.

Because this energy-producing process is complicated, it needs to be controlled. In our make-believe world of the cell city, control is achieved using methods like those of our real cities; a bureaucracy rules. Let's look at this bureaucracy.

The bureaucrats resemble each other closely. Their fellow rulers call them Robert, Alexander, and William (their exaggerated sense of importance allows no nicknames). They are pudgy, pompous, and per-snickety—and good administrators as long as everything is going well. However, any disruption causes disaster. You see, they are a tad slow in their thinking, a mite short on creativity, and a bit lacking in flexibility. The bureaucracy of the cell city is unlike that of our modern society, where flexibility, creativity, and clear thinking are so necessary and practical.

An old expression tells us that into every life a little rain must fall. Unfortunately for our bureaucrats, rain can turn into a flood. The problem arises from another group that populates our little cell city—a group of rebels.

Markedly different from the bureaucrats, as youngsters this second group went by the nicknames of Sly, Speed, and Flash; their names fit their mischief.

As adults they are fast-thinking, creative, and flexible, but lacking in responsibility. Their delight and pleasure in life is to torment the bureaucrats, and they know a perfect way to achieve this fiendish goal. You see, this fantastic energy production can work only if the fuel—which is hot and corrosive—is slowly and precisely transported to the furnaces (one of the few virtues of the bureaucrats is their slowness and precision). Our rebels delight in sending extra trainloads of fuel to the furnaces, where they dump it all over the floor.

You can imagine what happens next. Our poor bureaucrats, faced with this mess, call out the National Guard and enlist workers from factories and offices to shovel up the corrosive goo. This makes everybody unhappy. The National Guard is grumpy because the gooey fuel eats through their shiny boots. The office and factory workers hate the backbreaking work and their union strikes in protest, closing the assembly lines, supermarkets, and sales organizations of the little cell city. The city grinds to a halt, the voters complain, the mayor screams, the bureaucrats scurry about in quivering ineptness. It's a real mess.

Pity the poor bureaucrats. Slow-thinking, lacking creativity and flexibility, they are unprepared for this major disaster. They slowly and ploddingly restore the energy-producing system to normal and restart the offices and factories. And calm the mayor and soothe the voters. And wait for the next onslaught of excess fuel for the furnaces.

Perhaps you think the story of the little cell city is preposterous. If you do, you are wrong.

The marvelous material that stores the energy of the atom without the dangers of its radioactivity is sugar. The analogy of the furnaces is a good one; sugar slowly releases its fantastic energy, a bit at a time, as if it were traveling from furnace to furnace. In biochemistry books this process is called the Krebs cycle or the tricarboxylic acid cycle.

The counterparts of the bureaucrats in the body are the enzymes that precisely regulate sugar's energy release. Made of proteins, they regulate and assist in the splitting of the sugar molecule that releases energy. Without them, sugar would need the heat of a real furnace to split, making life impossible unless we were built like a home furnace.

So the furnacelike production of energy actually takes place in the body; because it is regulated by enzymes, there is no need for furnace heat. Enzymes do fantastic work, but don't be fooled. They are not creative or flexible or quick-thinking; they ploddingly and persistently perform the limited tasks to which they are assigned.

To continue the explanation, you must accept the rest of the story as I see it and as I believe it to be true.

It is tempting to look at our modern world, to see computers, bullet trains, and swept-wing fighter planes, and to conclude that not only has the world changed, but also that we've changed, that we have become as efficient as our machines. In some ways, perhaps we have—but not our bodies, not our cells.

The last thousand years have brought profound changes in our lifestyle. However, we have not changed. A thousand years is a tiny moment in the evolution of our bodies, of our cells. They are the same cells our ancestors possessed in the ancient past, in a cave, crowded close to a fire. In fact, they are not much changed from that monkeylike creature whose descendants walked upright and learned to talk. We share the same nutrition needs, digestion limits, and energy production method.

Although we have not changed, our diet has changed, specifically our use of refined foods. Prior to modern agriculture, foods were made of unrefined starch, protein, and fat.

Starches are made of individual sugar molecules, tightly bound together like links on a chain. In natural digestion the individual sugars are snapped off the chain slowly and ploddingly, allowing lots of time to process each sugar and insert it only when needed into the energy production system, the various furnaces. No hurry, everything orderly, everything natural. The bureaucratic control of energy is content.

Like starches, proteins are chains, and the chains are individual amino acids. These individual amino acids are broken off the chain slowly, ploddingly, and contentedly. As with starches, this natural process allows amino acids to be presented to the body only when needed.

But conditions change when industry, instead of the body, manufacture foods, a process called refining. Refining starches produces regrettable consequences. It breaks the bonds between sugar molecules so the sugar you eat and drink enters the stomach no longer as intact chains. The molecules are like the links of a broken chain; they are free. The body gobbles up this unchained sugar like a hungry shark in a goldfish aquarium.

Unfortunately, although our digestive system can regulate its intake of sugar from starch, it poorly regulates its intake of refined sugar. Conditioned by millions of years of evolution to handle a diet of starches, its enzymes do not have the flexibility and the creativity to adequately handle the flood of free sugar.

This refined sugar floods the body, causing the various systems that process sugar to overload. What happens then is unclear, although I like my fanciful explanation of the little cell city and the havoc that overload causes.

Before ending this section, a word about proteins. The story is much the same as with sugar. Refining breaks apart the linked amino acids that make protein. The free amino acids gush into the body, overwhelming the amino-acid-handling systems. The body suffers.

In MALS food allergy, there is no police force to exhaust. Someday, when we find the root cause, I believe it will be in our enzyme systems, enzymes needed to process these food chemicals. We will find these enzymes defective or missing. We trigger the immune system to launch the symptoms caused by food allergy when we eat more of these chemicals than we can process.

We have discussed several factors that can start us reacting to foods. One is genetic; allergy is written in our genes, the packets of information in our cells that determine who we are and that have such influence over how we react to the allergens in our environment. A second factor may be overwhelming environmental exposure to mite or mold—the unemployed mother unable to move her family from a moldy basement apartment.

There is one further reason beyond genetics and exposure why we suffer from food allergy.

Today we live long past the twenties and thirties that Mother Nature originally designed to be our old age. She can no longer discard us so easily. We fooled her. But it's not right to fool Mother Nature—she will have her revenge. And part of her revenge is our food allergy.

When we lived short lives, our numbers were small, and we suffered none of the diseases of old age—our short lives prevented these diseases. Our diet included foods gathered from forests, plains, and jungles, including edible roots, bulbs, and fruits. Above all, it included meat and animal products: the eggs and young birds we found in the trees, the animals we hunted, and the carrion we robbed from predators and other scavengers.

These days are gone. We have successfully extended our years of life and populated the land. We are no longer a small number of powerless humans; we are many. We no longer live the life for which nature designed us, the life of the hunter-gatherer; we would starve if we did. To survive in our millions, we learned to grow and manufacture food in abundance.

However, we lack variability in our diet. This lack of variability applies especially to classic food allergy. The foods we grow, raise, and eat in abundance tend to be only a few, such as milk, corn, wheat, and meat. They make up a large and unchanging part of our diets. However, Mother Nature not only made us meat eaters, over our millions of years of evolution she also made us eaters of foods of great variety. As our ancestors scrambled from branch to branch in the forest and roamed the plains where we evolved, we ate a variety of available meats, fruits, and berries. We ate anything we could get our hands on. Variability in our diet was further enhanced as different seasons provided different foods.

We ate insects, animals, roots, bulbs, and tubers. We ate when we found foods and did not eat if we found none. Our diets changed day by day and season by season. Because our diets varied so greatly, Mother Nature programmed our immune systems to demand a varied diet.

Little did she suspect that someday we would eat our modern diet, a diet with little variety. We consume wheat, corn, milk, and citrus fruits every day, often at every meal. Prepared by millions of years of evolution to function well on a diet of great variability, our immune systems weaken on this unvarying diet.

Let's return to our immune police force and look at the strains this unvarying diet imposes on them. In the station, the police that used to stop allergic reactions to the insects, roots, and tubers find little to do. Our intake of these foods is small.

Other police are swamped with work. The wheat, milk, citrus, and corn police no sooner stop our immune reaction against these foods at one meal than they must rush into the bloodstream all over again. The next meal contains the same foods. They never find time to rest.

If you do not suffer from food allergy, this constant diet does not bother your immune system. We who suffer food reactions are not so fortunate; our food police become weak and exhausted from the constant struggle. They can no longer defend against food allergy. They can no longer stop the senseless immune attack on the foods we eat daily. We suffer headaches, tiredness, stomach pain, and other miserable symptoms.

To help relieve classic food allergy, our immune systems need a break from this monotonous diet, a day off once in a while. That's why varying your diet can work so well. Not eating wheat, corn, milk, or citrus fruits for a day gives the police responsible for these foods a well-deserved respite—a chance to refresh themselves. Then, when you return to eating these foods again, your refreshed immune police can stop your immune system from attacking the foods. Alternatively, they gain this rest if we eat only a small amount of the food each day, an amount they can easily control.

Is this police force a figment of my imagination? No; it exists. The police I described are cells of the immune system, cells called lymphocytes. The lymphocytes that stop allergic reactions are called suppresser lymphocytes, and, as their name indicates, they suppress or stop allergic reactions to foods. When they weaken, when they become exhausted, we suffer the immediate or delayed symptoms of food protein allergy.

As classic food allergy is affected by our modern diet, so is MALS food allergy. We owe our current diet high in refined sugar, acid, MSG, and low-calorie sweeteners to modern agriculture and our desire for a delicious meal. Although we must be proud of scientific farming—without it, modern society is impossible—we also need to regret the allergic illness it spawns. Truly, we fooled Mother Nature, but on those of us who suffer food allergy, she takes her revenge.

CHAPTER 4

Syndromes of Food Allergy

Classic and MALS Food Allergies: Mild Immediate Symptoms

Now is the time to concentrate more intently on food allergy symptoms caused by these two food allergies, and we will do so in this chapter. These symptoms often follow definite patterns; when they do so, they are called syndromes, and I will point them out as I mention them.

Immediate but Mild Symptoms Caused by Classic and MALS Food Allergies

As we discussed, both food allergies cause both delayed symptoms and symptoms that arise quickly after we eat. We call the quickly appearing symptoms "immediate" symptoms; the name accurately describes how quickly symptoms begin: within minutes after eating even a tiny amount of troublesome food.

You may think that you can easily recognize symptoms that start while you eat a food or shortly afterward. You are right—in the case of severe symptoms. You may be startled by a dramatic shortness of breath or feel miserable with your skin covered with terribly itchy hives. You cannot ignore these symptoms. However, this same ease of recognition may not exist in the case of mild symptoms. They can fool you, and you can miss them because they may appear as a dimly noticed uneasiness, a mild distress, a vague discomfort. You may pay them no attention, and the food bothering you may escape your notice.

To search for these mild reactions, medical professionals often use tests. Using these tests—whether performed on blood or on the skin— mild immediate classic food allergies most easily reveal themselves.

However, too often when symptoms are mild, doctors and patients can misinterpret what the tests tell them. They must be interpreted with caution. We will examine these tests and see why caution is necessary when we try to interpret them.

(As we discussed, the tests do not show delayed classic or MALS food allergies unless the medical care professional designs the tests to show these allergies.)

Skin, Blood, and Other Tests
to Diagnose Food Allergy

In my patients with classic food allergy, I frequently see evidence of mild symptoms that appear quickly after eating. Many of my patients who react quickly show positive results to foods when we test their skin, and these results often surprise them. The same is true in blood tests that often show this same food allergy, even in patients who fail to realize that they are allergic to foods.

To understand how this happens, it helps to briefly review a topic we covered when we discussed the cause of classic food allergy. Now we can apply this information to help us understand some of the results we find when we perform skin and blood tests.

I believe that all of us are allergic to the proteins of foods. We share this allergy whether the foods we eat make us sick or if we eat them with no ill effects whatsoever. Our allergy comes courtesy of our immune systems. These systems continually hunt for germs by searching for any strange foreign protein in our bloodstream that may betray the presence of a germ. When they find this strange protein, they attack.

These proteins gain entrance to our bloodstreams when we eat a food such as shrimp or peanut. Then, our immune systems find it and launch a full-scale attack, bringing on sneezing, wheezing, itching, and abdominal cramps in allergic people.

In nonallergic people, this mistaken attack on innocent food protein stops quickly. A regulator in the immune system decides that the attack is silly and quickly stops the attack. Although the regulator cannot prevent us from being allergic to food protein, it prevents our immune systems from making us suffer from this allergy.

Because we are all allergic to foods, finding this allergy on skin or blood tests should not surprise us. Nor should we think that the tests are trying to tell us that we will react severely to these foods. In those who suffer little or not at all from allergy, eating the food will cause mild or no discomfort.

But if we are all allergic to food protein, why do only some of us suffer when we eat the food? Because we who react to food have a weak regulator. It cannot stop the attack or prevent the symptoms the attack causes. How much we suffer from this reaction depends on how sensitive we are to foods.

Our symptoms of food allergy are not all the same; they vary in intensity as much as humans vary in weight. Some of us react to certain foods as if we were hit by a three-hundred-pound football lineman, battered with debilitating headaches and explosive diarrhea. Others suffer symptoms so mild we do not notice them or dismiss them as of little consequence.

If our food allergy is of the mild variety, we can eat the foods without trouble. Although our blood or skin test shows allergy, it is no big deal. However, if our symptoms more resemble battering from the lineman, quickly appearing pain and discomfort alert us to the troublesome food.

Therefore, whether we notice our allergy to the foods that show positive results on tests depends on the way we react to them. Not all positive skin or blood tests mean severe food allergy.

You may suffer mild food allergy and be unaware of your allergy. Soon after you eat peanuts or popcorn, you may experience a vague discomfort. Perhaps your nose feels a little stuffy, or the skin on your face and arms itches. Your stomach may feel somewhat crampy, with mildly uncomfortable pressure.

You may feel a lump in your throat after drinking milk or orange juice. Perhaps you must work harder to breathe, and your breath wheezes out of your chest. Immediate MALS or classic food allergy can cause all of these symptoms; if the symptoms bother you little, you can easily overlook your food allergy.

Jim is a good example of a person with mild immediate food allergy.

Jim came to see us because he suffers sneezing, wheezing, and red eyes from spring and fall pollen. We just finished skin-testing him and recorded the huge hives that signal a positive test to oak and ragweed pollen. Since oak trees release their pollen in spring and ragweed plants release their pollen in fall, these tests correspond well with his story of spring and fall hay fever.

How about the large hives that formed at the peanut and cabbage test sites? Jim did not mention allergy to them in his story. In fact, Jim is questioning them. He asks, "I've never noticed any trouble with these foods. Is the skin test wrong?"

That's possible but unlikely. To understand why, it helps to know that although the skin tests identify food allergies, they do not tell us if the allergies are mild or severe. They will show as large a hive to mildly troubling foods as they do to foods that cause life-threatening symptoms.

It's easy to be led astray by these positive skin tests if you believe that the test identifies only major allergies that you must avoid at all costs. When your allergy to foods is slight, the positive tests can confuse you when you find you can eat these foods.

Just because peanut and cabbage show a positive reaction does not mean you must banish them from the diet. If your allergy is mild, you can eat them without harm. Or they may cause mild discomfort if you eat too much of them, but you can avoid this discomfort by limiting their intake to the amount you tolerate well.

From Jim we learn that a positive skin test to food does not always mean a severe food allergy. Many of our patients have these minimally troublesome food allergies; you may have them, too.

In Jim's case, since peanut and cabbage allergy bother him little, are they unimportant? No; I suspect they are very important at times. To explain this answer, let me tell you about my experience with pollen sufferers like Jim.

We treat many patients who suffer severe pollen allergy. Early in my practice I noticed that while some patients received great relief from treatment with a continuous series of pollen injections to reduce their allergy to pollen, some did not—they continued to suffer. Terrible sneezing and itchy eyes made the tiny pollen floating on the delightful summer breezes instruments of torture.

Hay Fever and Mild Immediate Food Allergy

Like Jim, many of my hay fever patients showed unexpected positive food skin tests. Once we discovered their food allergy and they avoided or limited their intake of these foods during the pollen seasons, they felt much better. Our treatment failures decreased, and I was delighted.

Therefore, even mild immediate food allergy, whether MALS or classic, becomes important in certain circumstances—when a person is overwhelmed by exposure to a strong allergen such as pollen. Then, even though the food allergy is mild, it still worsens the suffering. The same foods eaten with impunity in winter's cold air can bring punishing distress in summer's warmth.

That's why we told Jim to beware of peanuts and cabbage when his sneezing and wheezing begin.

Other Allergies and Mild Immediate Classic or MALS Food Allergies

Hay fever is not the only allergic illness worsened by coexisting mild immediate food allergy. Patients who live with a cat or a dog often suffer increased symptoms if they eat certain foods that cause no symptoms when they are not exposed to animals. Many of our patients who are suffering from hives experience unbearable itching if they eat certain foods that they eat without trouble after their hives disappear.

To restate these thoughts: when people with immediate food allergy are reacting to pollen, pet dander, or other allergies, they often lose the ability to easily tolerate the foods that cause little or no trouble at less stressful times.

Do You Need a Test to Find These Mild Immediate Food Allergies?

You do not need tests to find these mild immediate food allergies. If you suffer no symptoms, forget about these allergies. They are not hurting you, so why bother?

However, think about mild food allergies during times when you react to another allergy. If you suffer greatly from cats or ragweed pollen, watch what you eat when you are exposed to cats or ragweed pollen. Do your cat or ragweed symptoms worsen when you eat certain foods such as peanuts or cabbage? Or oranges and tomatoes? If so, avoid these foods during the ragweed season or when you are exposed to cats.

If you do not have access to tests for allergy to foods, you should be able to identify them. Just keep these mild food allergies in mind and watch for them during times of allergic stress.

Not all immediate food symptoms are mild. Some strike far more severely, and some are even dangerous. To explore this danger, we will next look at the most flagrant form of immediate food allergy, anaphylaxis, an awkward word that in Greek means "without guarding." As the name indicates, this dangerous event happens suddenly, without warning, and without a chance for the affected person to guard against it.

Anaphylaxis: The Dangerous Food Reaction

Don't let the word "anaphylaxis" (an uh fa *lack* sis) intimidate you, but realize that experiencing anaphylaxis will. If you suffer from it, you will be frightened. Your symptoms will appear suddenly, usually within seconds to minutes. In about a third of cases, the symptoms subside and then restart one to three hours later, and these later symptoms can be as dangerous as the quick-appearing symptoms.

Anaphylaxis can affect your skin, your intestines, your blood vessels and heart, or your breathing passages. If it affects your skin, you may feel aggravating skin itching and heat, and you may notice a red flush over parts of your body and even see the welts of hives appear on your skin. If it affects your intestines, you may suffer vomiting, painful cramps, gas, or bloating, which can progress to diarrhea.

Most forms of anaphylaxis bring only mild and nonthreatening symptoms. A few hives, a little stomach cramp. Only a few are dangerous. The most dangerous symptoms fall into two main categories: those that affect your breathing, and those that threaten to send you into shock.

Anaphylaxis can threaten any part of your breathing passages. For instance, after eating a peanut or a shrimp, the first part of your breathing passages, your nose, may drip copious amounts of fluid or close off so tightly that you cannot move air through it.

Your tongue may swell so large that it forces your mouth open; that little projection that hangs down at the back of your mouth, the uvula, may swell right into your throat, partly blocking your breathing, gagging you, and interfering with your swallowing. Your voice may turn hoarse.

The same swelling farther along the air passages—from your throat to deep in your chest—may make you feel that your breath is being choked off, and you may wheeze. If the swelling anywhere along your breathing passages progresses farther, you may not be able to breathe at all.

If your blood pressure drops after eating peanuts or tree nuts, you may feel dizzy, faint, and confused. If your blood pressure drops farther, you may experience even more severe dizziness and—even more dangerous—you may fall unconscious. If your blood pressure continues to drop, you may slip into shock from which you do not recover.

How Dangerous Is Anaphylaxis?

For those struck by this frightening reaction, the danger is real. The figures are not precise, but between one hundred and five hundred people die of anaphylaxis each year. We need to fear this threatening reaction, but we also need to put its danger in perspective.

Foods do not cause all anaphylactic deaths. Stings from insects such as bees or wasps cause many of these deaths. Drugs, including ordinary pain medications such as aspirin, contribute their own grim statistics. Foods cause only a small percentage of these anaphylactic deaths.

How many? A number of studies of emergency room visits for anaphylaxis indicate that foods cause about third of these reactions, with insect stings and medication allergies combining to cause about another third. Of those few who died, peanuts and tree nuts were the most frequent causes.

The people most at risk for near-fatal or fatal reactions to foods are those with asthma, a great risk factor; also, those who had suffered food anaphylaxis before, especially those who ate a food containing a nut or a peanut that made them react in the past.

As for your own risk of an anaphylactic reaction to foods, it is minor. Only a small percentage of allergic people will ever experience anaphylaxis; of these few, only a very small number find their lives in danger.

If you have never experienced this food allergy symptom, your chance of suffering a life-threatening anaphylactic reaction to food is probably equivalent to your chance of being hit by lightning. Nevertheless, as you should not run around in a lightning storm carrying a metal rod, so you should not underestimate this scary allergic reaction. If you react to a food quickly and severely, avoid it.

Mild Anaphylaxis

Less severe anaphylactic reactions to foods are far more common then severe reactions; they scare you but do not threaten you. You may feel a little stuffiness, a little breathing difficulty, a little dizzy. From my experiences with allergic patients, these minor anaphylactic reactions happen surprisingly often.

You may experience these symptoms now; they could start tomorrow, next year, or ten years from now. Because foods may cause these symptoms, you should be aware of this problem. Forewarned is forearmed.

Which Foods Cause Anaphylaxis?

I reviewed the studies on anaphylaxis to find the foods that trip it off.

FOODS MENTIONED IN STUDIES ON FOOD-INDUCED ANAPHYLAXIS

Most Commonly Implicated

Crustaceans (include lobster, crab, shrimp)

Peanuts

Less Commonly Implicated
(order of importance unknown)

Avocado

Banana

Celery

Cereal grains

Egg

Fish

Garlic

Kiwi

Legumes other than peanuts (soy, peas, lentils, guar gum)

Milk

Papaya

Seeds

Tree nuts (e.g., almonds, Brazil nuts, cashews, filberts, and pecans)

Wheat

Of the above foods, peanut, tree nut, fish, and shellfish allergies are likely to last a lifetime. Cow's milk, egg, and cereal grain allergies are likely to disappear with time, if they occur in infants. If allergies occur later in life, the chances of outgrowing them is far less.

This list does not include all the foods that cause anaphylaxis. In susceptible people, almost any food may cause this frightening reaction, including foods with large amounts of the MALS chemicals.

Unknown Causes of Anaphylaxis

In each of the studies I reviewed, the cause of the anaphylactic reaction remained unknown in 30 percent to 40 percent of cases. I strongly suspect that many of these reactions arose from the refined sugar, acid foods, low-calorie sweeteners, or MSG that are part of the MALS food allergy.

We have discussed how MALS and classic food allergies trigger off the same symptoms. In my practice I have seen many patients treated in the emergency room for threatening reactions, but the doctors who treated them could not determine the cause. In most cases, eliminating MSG prevented future reactions. If the doctors who studied these anaphylactic reactions had realized the importance of the MALS chemicals and searched for their tracks, I believe that the percentage of unknown causes would have shrunk dramatically.

Fortunately, people affected by classic food allergy tend to react to only one or a few foods. When they find and avoid these foods, they no longer suffer anaphylaxis. Patients with MALS food allergy are not so fortunate; they must avoid many foods that contain high levels of MALS food chemicals, especially MSG.

Avoiding and Treating Anaphylaxis

Avoiding and treating anaphylaxis means using your good common sense. Some of the measures you should follow include:

◊ Watch to see which foods cause your anaphylaxis.
◊ If you are unsure of the foods that cause your reaction, ask your medical care professional to help you identify them.
◊ Be cautious of MSG, low-calorie sweeteners, sugary foods, and acidic foods—they may cause or worsen your reactions.

◊ If you know that you react severely to wheat, milk, peanuts, shrimp, or other foods, remove them completely from your diet.

◊ Always carry emergency medicine including, at a minimum, an injection of epinephrine. Quick treatment with epinephrine is life-saving. Seek skilled emergency help if you experience an anaphylactic reaction.

◊ Aspirinlike pain medications cause anaphylaxis in some people. Avoid these pain medications if you have ever experienced anaphylaxis.

◊ Beta-blocker medications may make treating anaphylaxis more difficult. Check with your doctor about their use.

◊ Do not become complacent. All allergies can appear intermittently. If you once suffered a reaction, it can happen again. It may even be caused by foods you have repeatedly eaten without trouble. Eternal vigilance is often the price of survival.

◊ If you suffer anaphylactic reaction to foods, join The Food Allergy Network, an organization dedicated to food-sensitive people. Contact:

> The Food Allergy Network
> 10400 Eaton Place, Suite 107
> Fairfax, VA 22030-2208
> Fax: (703) 691-2713
> Phone: (800) 929-4040
> Phone outside of United States: (703) 691-3179
> www.foodallergy.org

You may suffer a special and confusing type of anaphylaxis. Called exercise anaphylaxis, this reaction takes place where you would never expect it. Let's look at this mysterious affliction next.

Exercise-Induced Anaphylaxis

A discussion about anaphylaxis would be incomplete without mentioning this strange immediate food reaction. It happens only while a person exercises; it torments the poor, unsuspecting exercisers who perspire to promote health. Instead of gaining muscle tone, they experience a reaction that, when severe, threatens to end not only their health but also their life.

Picture the poor jogger, already suffering near misses from heedless drivers, wet by dripping skies and bit by yipping dogs. To these travails add one more unpleasant experience—exercise anaphylaxis. Jogging is not the only activity that precipitates exercise anaphylaxis; any hard exercise can cause it. If you are affected, you may develop the typical symptoms of anaphylaxis as you dig up your garden, pump iron, or run up and down stairs cleaning the house.

Symptoms You May Experience

Symptoms can be the same as we noted in our look at anaphylaxis that occurs without exercise. Following your morning run, you may notice a warm sensation that spreads all over your body. Perhaps you next notice itching—an annoying itching that starts in your scalp and extends to your big toe. Then you notice big red hives pop out on your arms; hurrying to a mirror, you notice one prominent one on your nose and another covering your right ear, leaving it red and swollen.

If your reaction is mild, nothing more may happen. However, if your reaction worsens, your symptoms may turn from simply annoying to positively frightening. The hives migrate into your breathing passages, making you wheeze and gasp for breath. They may swell up in your intestine, bringing you painful abdominal cramps as your intestine tries fruitlessly to squeeze the swelling away.

If the exercise anaphylaxis worsens further, it may completely block your breathing. It may drop your blood pressure, making you weak, dizzy, and close to shock. It may even disrupt your heart's rhythm, giving you a frightening feeling that your heart is missing beats, that it is stopping and starting most alarmingly.

From mild to severe, these are symptoms of exercise anaphylaxis.

Searching for the Bad Foods

You may find great difficulty identifying the foods that cause your exercise anaphylaxis. They could be foods you ate hours before your exercise, and this prolonged interval between eating and suffering may cloud the cause/effect relationship.

The thought that a food caused your reaction may not even cross your mind. But it should; foods often cause this reaction, and they are the same ones that cause the anaphylaxis I mentioned in the previous section, anaphylaxis that happens without exercise.

Further masking the guilty food, you may have eaten many foods in the hours before you exercised. Thus, even if you know that foods caused your reaction, you may be unsure of the food or foods responsible.

Which Foods Cause Exercise Anaphylaxis?

The best way to find the food or foods that cause your exercise anaphylaxis is by being suspicious of the foods that cause ordinary anaphylaxis. To help you remember them, I listed some of them below:

FOODS MENTIONED IN STUDIES ON EXERCISE ANAPHYLAXIS

Most Commonly Implicated

Crustaceans (include lobster, crab, shrimp)

Peanuts

Less Commonly Implicated*
(order of frequency unknown)

Avocado

Banana

Celery

Cereal grains

Egg

Fish

Garlic

Kiwi

Legumes other than peanuts (soy, peas, lentils, guar gum)

Milk

Papaya

Seeds

Tree nuts (e.g., almonds, Brazil nuts, cashews, filberts, and pecans)

Wheat

* Any food can cause exercise anaphylaxis in susceptible people.

In addition to this list, foods high in the MALS chemicals also cause exercise anaphylaxis.

Now that you know some of the foods to suspect, start making lists. List all the foods you have eaten in the twenty-four hours prior to your reaction. The next time it happens, list the foods you ate in the twenty-four hours prior to that reaction. Foods that appear on both lists become automatic suspects.

How to Avoid Exercise Anaphylaxis

You can take the following steps to help protect yourself from this worrisome food reaction. We have already covered many of these suggestions, and I will repeat them here:

◊ Be careful exercising during extremely hot or cold weather, during your allergy season, or in humid weather.

◊ If you are unsure of the foods that cause your reaction, ask your medical care provider to help you identify them.

◊ If you suspect MALS food allergy, do not eat MSG or low-calorie sweetener-containing foods for twenty-four hours before hard exercise. Avoid sugary and acidic foods for twelve hours before exercise.

◊ If you know that wheat, milk, peanuts, shrimp, or other foods caused your past anaphylaxis, remove them completely from your diet. Do this even if you plan to spend the day vegetating on the couch in front of the TV set. Why take a chance that you will participate in an unplanned exercise that will trip off another attack?

◊ If you do not know which foods cause your anaphylaxis, do not exercise. Alternatively, fast for at least four and preferably six hours before you exercise. This is not a foolproof measure; anaphylaxis can occur more than four hours after the food is eaten, although there is some suggestion that most of the reactions occur in the first four hours.

◊ Do not exercise if you have eaten any suspect foods within the past twelve hours.

◊ Always carry emergency medicine including, at a minimum, an injection of epinephrine. Never jog or do other hard exercise without it.

◇ If you engage in any hard exercise such as jogging, always have a friend accompany you who is able to give you emergency aid, especially the epinephrine.

◇ At the first sign that a reaction is starting, stop exercise immediately and seek skilled emergency help.

◇ Start any exercise program slowly; you may be able to avoid anaphylaxis by gradually increasing the exercise until your body adjusts to it.

◇ Some people experience anaphylaxis from aspirinlike pain medications. Avoid their use. Beta-blocker medications may prime you for a reaction and interfere with treating it. Check with your doctor to see if your medicine includes a beta-blocker.

◇ Join The Food Allergy Network.

◇ Do not become complacent. All allergies, including exercise anaphylaxis, can appear intermittently. If you once suffered a reaction, it can happen again, even after repeated exercise without anaphylaxis. Eternal vigilance is often the price of survival.

Why Make a Big Deal of a Rare Reaction?

Severe forms of exercise anaphylaxis bother few of us, but mild forms bother many of us; they are not so rare. You may be affected, so you should know about this odd food allergy symptom.

Be Alert for Minor Forms of Anaphylaxis

Because our lesser symptoms never approach the enormity of a flagrant reaction, we often fail to realize that we suffer a minor form of exercise anaphylaxis. When jogging makes our noses run or our intestines hurt, we do not think of immediate food allergy. When we dig up the garden or play tennis and our skin itches, our chest hurts, or we run out of breath quickly, we do not think about what we ate for lunch two hours ago. When our hearts miss a beat or two or we feel a lump in our chest that blocks our breathing, we remain unaware that we suffer from a small anaphylactic reaction.

I told you about the small and full-grown forms of anaphylaxis so you will understand your own symptoms better. With this understanding you can search for and find the food or foods provoking your attacks and take it or them out of your diet. Eliminating such food stops the reaction and helps you find the good health you deserve. Good health comes only to those prepared by knowledge to receive it.

There are other forms of immediate food allergies that you should know about, and we will cover them next.

Special Types of Immediate Allergy to Foods

You should know about two conditions of immediate food allergy that may affect you or a member of your family. The first involves food allergy that coexists with allergy to a component of rubber called latex. The second involves a contact allergy to foods. Both are classic food allergies; they do not involve the MALS foods.

Latex Sensitivity

Rubber is everywhere. I find it difficult to visualize our modern society without rubber. How would our underpants or bras stay on without the elastic support of rubber? Picture yourself carrying around stacks of cards without those ever-useful rubber bands. Or trying to bounce a ball made, not of springy rubber, but of unyielding plastic. Or blowing up a balloon made of paper. The cards would fall, the ball would thud on the floor, and the balloon would burst. You would be frustrated.

Rubber is everywhere and is ever useful. However, we pay a price for this essential of modern civilization: allergy to rubber.

Many plants produce the rubber that we find so useful. The milk-weed plant makes rubber. You see it oozing as a milky liquid from the injured plant. You notice it bleeding from the wound of a cut poppy. It also leaks from cuts in the rubber tree; rubber workers make these cuts and harvest the liquid to make the commercial rubber products we use every day.

The rubber they collect is a complex material made up of many components. The component that causes allergy is called latex. Anyone can become allergic to latex, and this possibility increases if you work in certain occupations that expose you to repeated contact with rubber. For example, if you work in the rubber manufacturing business, you are heavily exposed. Health care workers also are heavily exposed through the rubber gloves they wear. Up to 20 percent of nurses, hospital housekeepers, and operating room personnel suffer rubber latex allergy, an allergy also shared by their patients who undergo repeated operations that subject them to intimate exposure to rubber in gloves, tubes, and other medical implements.

Local and Systemic Allergies to Latex

In general, latex-sensitive people show their allergy to this substance in two ways, locally and systemically. As the name implies, local allergies strike the area touched by latex and do not spread far from this area. The reaction stays localized. Systemic allergies range far outside the area of contact; they are carried by the blood vessel system to any part of the body.

Symptoms of local allergy. If you suffer a local allergy to latex, you may feel your hands swelling as you don rubber gloves. They swell because the rubber touches your hands, leaving molecules of latex where it touches your skin—your skin swells as it reacts to these molecules. As another example, your mouth and lips may itch where they touched rubber balloons as you helped your child inflate them for her party. Another sign: you may develop an itchy rash where the exposed elastic in your underpants touches your skin.

With this exposure to latex, your skin itches and turns red. You continually scratch your itchy skin and this scratching thickens the skin and dries it out. Continued scratching further irritates your skin, making it crack and bleed.

Not all local reactions are caused by latex. You may react not to the latex component of the rubber product, but to other chemicals that remain after the rubber manufacturing processes are finished. This contact reaction will give you a local rash much like the local rash caused by latex.

Symptoms of systemic allergy. A systemic allergy carries far greater danger than a local allergy. These symptoms usually arise from the latex clinging to the powder of powdered latex gloves. Nonpowdered latex gloves do not seem to cause systemic reactions.

These symptoms could be many: your nose may stuff up and drip fluid. You may wheeze and find yourself straining to expel the breath from your lungs; hives may make your skin itch and swell, even in areas never touched by latex.

In some people the reaction progresses to dangerous, full-blown anaphylaxis, with breathing blockage, shock, and for an unfortunate few, danger of death. Truly, a systemic reaction to latex must not be lightly dismissed.

Latex Allergy and Immediate Reactions to Foods
Why discuss latex allergy in a book on food allergy? Because the people who react to latex with immediate systemic reactions such as anaphylaxis can suffer the same reactions to food.

This may sound surprising, but a little background information shows that it really isn't. The information involves the protein in latex and the laziness of Mother Nature.

Latex allergy is directed against the protein of rubber. The day Mother Nature made this protein, she was lazy. Instead of inventing all-new and unique proteins for latex, she used some of the same proteins she used to make other plants, the same proteins she placed in the fruits, vegetables, nuts, and seeds you eat daily.

If you are allergic to latex, you may suffer the consequences of Mother Nature's laziness: you may also react to the proteins in certain foods that are shared by latex. This is classic food allergy at work and leads to the following summary and caution:

If you work with rubber, use rubber gloves in your work, or have undergone repeated surgical procedures, you may react to latex. Even if you belong to none of the above categories, you still may react to latex. If so, you may also suffer if you eat foods that share latex's protein. Watch for symptoms when you eat these foods and avoid them if they cause you distress.

Alternatively, if you react to the foods I mention below, beware of a simultaneous allergy to latex.

Which Foods Are Involved
Many of the foods listed on page 184 are known to share proteins with latex. They may cause symptoms in the latex-sensitive person.

Who knows how long this list may become as other foods that share latex proteins join the list in the future? For the present, you can use this list. If you react to these foods, beware of latex sensitivity. If you react to latex, beware of allergy to these foods. However, do not stop eating them unless you notice that you react to them. Why remove perfectly harmless foods from your diet? Also, do not use powdered latex gloves or be around people who use them.

FOODS TO WHICH THE LATEX-SENSITIVE
PERSON MAY REACT*

Fruits	Vegetables	Seeds/Nuts
Apple	Avocado	Chestnut
Apricot	Carrot	Fennel seed
Banana	Celery	Hazelnut (filbert)
Cantaloupe	Parsley	Sunflower seed
Cherry	Potato	
Fig	Tomato	
Honeydew		
Kiwi		
Mango		
Orange		
Papaya		
Peach		
Pear		
Pineapple		
Watermelon		

*Other foods not mentioned here may also affect the latex-sensitive person.

The Oral Allergy Syndrome

Doctors noticed this syndrome relatively recently. The name describes it well. People with oral allergy syndrome suffer uncomfortable mouths, gums, lips, tongues, and throats when they eat certain fresh fruits and vegetables.

If you suffer this distressing food allergy, you may notice discomfort starting while you eat a fresh apple. As you chew, the apple juice and pulp fill your mouth, also touching your gums, lips, tongue, and throat. Where they touch, you feel an aggravating itchiness. An equally irritating swelling quickly follows the itch, puffing up your tongue and lips. After some time—as you would expect with an immediate food allergy—the itch and swelling gradually fade.

All the structures in your mouth may be affected, or only one or two, such as the tongue, gums, or throat. You may react to only one fruit or to all the fresh fruits and vegetables you eat. How and to what you react depend on the way you react.

Is this allergy important? It is. The oral allergy syndrome affects more people than the food allergy associated with latex. I see the oral allergy syndrome frequently in my practice. It is a variety of classic food allergy.

The oral allergy syndrome often affects the people who suffer from hay fever—who sneeze, wheeze, and itch from breathing summer's pollen. Why are these hay fever sufferers affected? The answer is the same one we discussed in latex allergy: they suffer because Mother Nature is lazy.

In latex allergy, Mother Nature spares herself trouble by making latex out of many of the same proteins that she uses to make certain foods. She succumbed to the same laziness when she made fresh fruits and vegetables—she used some of the same proteins to make pollen. Therefore, people allergic to these shared proteins in pollen can also react to the same proteins in fresh fruits and vegetables.

The Involved Foods
Fresh fruits and vegetables cause the oral allergy syndrome. The word "fresh" must be stressed; only fresh fruits and vegetables cause this contact reaction. Any process that destroys freshness—such as canning or boiling—prevents the oral allergy syndrome.

People who suffer oral allergy syndrome from fresh cherries, peaches, apples, or other fruits and vegetables can eat them canned or boiled. They may also be able to eat fruits and vegetables that have been frozen.

Although affected people may suffer symptoms from any fresh fruit or vegetable, they more likely will react to certain foods if they suffer from certain pollen allergies. The table on page 186 points out these foods.

As you chew that delicious apple, your teeth release these proteins. As they fill your mouth, they contact your gums, lips, tongue, throat, and the inner lining of your mouth, setting off a hivelike itch and swelling. Once you degrade the protein by heat and perhaps freezing, you can eat the food without trouble.

FOODS TO WATCH IF YOU SUFFER FROM
THESE POLLEN ALLERGIES*

Spring Birch Pollen	Midsummer Grass Pollen	Fall Ragweed Pollen
Apples	Celery	Bananas
Carrots	Peach	Melons (watermelon, cantaloupe, honeydew)
Celery	Tomato	
Hazelnuts		Gourd family
Kiwi		(cucumber and
Peach		squash)
Potatoes		

*This is not an inclusive list. Further studies will find other relationships between foods and pollens.

Many patients are being treated with injections of pollen to reduce their summer hay fever sneezing, wheezing, and itchy eyes. A natural question is: Since allergy injections contain the proteins of pollen, and since many of these same proteins cause food allergy, will allergy injections lessen the impact of the oral allergy syndrome?

Studies show that they do, and in the section "Dealing with Your Immediate Food Allergy" we will look further at this treatment.

When Immediate Food Allergy Hides Deeply

We have discussed ways in which you can react to foods (syndromes of food allergy) such as anaphylaxis and the oral allergy syndrome. You should now recognize these syndromes if they affect you or a loved one. In a way, as they bring pain and discomfort, they also bring one benefit: their unmistakable symptoms point right to food allergy.

For example, if anaphylaxis strikes you, whether following your morning run or while relaxing at dinner, you now know that you must suspect MALS or classic food allergy. If your mouth swells with the oral allergy syndrome, you know that you must avoid certain fresh fruits and vegetables.

It is a pity that, as I mentioned, those who suffer from these recognizable syndromes of immediate food allergy occupy only the tip of our allergic iceberg. The majority of immediate food reactors do not suffer such easily recognized allergic reactions; we may not know that foods cause our distress.

At this time I will return to a subject we already covered in our discussion of mild food allergy: food allergy not suspected by the sufferer. I do this to reinforce in your mind that food allergy often is subtle in its signs but odious in its actions. You must watch for it.

Jim's hay fever symptoms go wild if he eats fresh fruits and vegetables in the fall; foods cause fits of sneezing and itching. He discovered this relationship between foods and pollen by himself, without any help from food allergy tests.

Not all patients are as observant as Jim is. Many fail to recognize these food/pollen relationships, and Marlene serves as a good example.

Marlene's skin tests are completed. They show huge reactions to pollens and similarly large reactions to foods.

Marlene looks at the test results and says, "Dr. Walsh, I expect to be allergic to the pollens because in the spring and fall my nose is stuffy and my headaches are horrible. The skin tests show these pollen allergies, as I expected. But I'm surprised that they also show reactions to foods, and these test reactions are large. I've never noticed that foods bother me. Are the food tests wrong?"

"I don't think so, Marlene," I reply. "Many of our patients suffer from hidden food allergies; I suspect you that you also suffer from hidden food allergies. Foods may be making your hay fever far worse than it needs to be. If we fail to search for these unsuspected food allergies, they would continue to make your summer hay fever unbearable and block the effects of our treatment."

I explained my comments by telling her about the example of the bucket of water.

Allergy and a Bucket of Water

We who are burdened by allergies must carry our load of symptom as if we were carrying a bucket of water. As long as our bucket is not over-filled with water, it won't overflow and splash all over us. If we add too much water to the bucket, we get wet.

We carry allergies like we carry water: we stay dry as long as we do not overfill our bucket. We overfill it by living in surroundings too musty for us or by reacting to the pollen-filled breezes on a warm summer day. Eating foods to which we have mild allergy further fills the bucket.

When we do this, when we overfill our bucket, our symptoms splash out, making us sneeze, wheeze, itch, and ache with headaches.

Both Jim and Marlene carry their buckets comfortably when the air is clear of pollen. While breathing no pollen, their food allergy fits comfortably in the bucket. It does not overflow. They suffer no food allergy symptoms.

However, when tree, grass, or ragweed pollens fill the air, they form part of the load in their allergy buckets, and hay fever symptoms splash out. With the bucket so loaded with pollen allergy, minor food allergies can no longer be carried easily. Foods that they eat without trouble the rest of the year now aggravate their sneezing, wheezing, itching, and headaches, these symptoms gushing forth like water pouring from an overfilled bucket.

Jim and Marlene's food allergies hide deep inside them, not emerging during low-allergy months. If I fail to warn them about these hidden food allergies, they will not avoid them. Their hay fever symptoms become so severe that our medications and allergy injections give poor relief.

Who Is Affected

Deeply hidden immediate food symptoms affect people who react quickly to their allergens, such as hay fever sufferers.

When people with these immediate reactors cuddle a cat, quickly their noses run, their eyes itch, and their skin turns red. They walk in the fall breezes, sniff their lovely fragrances, get a noseful of ragweed pollen, and sneeze convulsively. They eat a shrimp or a peanut, quickly break out in hives, and struggle to move air thorough their closing throats.

My patients' stories contain many other examples, but I think these examples reinforce my previous comments about how people suffering immediate symptoms from pollen and other allergens are susceptible to hidden immediate food symptoms.

Diagnosing Deeply Hidden Food Symptoms

Finding out if you suffer from deeply hidden food allergy may not be easy. If I would order blood tests on people who react quickly to the allergens, I will likely find high levels of the quick-reacting antibody called IgE in their blood if they are suffering from classic or food-protein allergy. This antibody reacts with the cat, ragweed pollen, shrimp, or peanut and causes these dramatic, uncomfortable, and at times dangerous allergy reactions.

Blood tests may miss these food symptoms, so you cannot rely on them to always point out the involved foods.

Skin tests often show hidden food allergies better than blood tests, but you may not have access to skin tests. Even with skin tests, you can miss this diagnosis; this food allergy often appears only on the injection (intradermal) part of the skin test. If your doctor does not perform injection tests, you may not learn about these foods, and even doctors, at times, miss this food allergy.

The food chemicals of MALS food allergy cause these same hidden food allergies. They cannot be identified by blood tests and are seldom looked for on skin tests.

Finding Hidden Food Allergies without Tests

Your best way to diagnose deeply hidden food allergies is to be alert to their possible presence. Consult with your medical caregiver. If you find yourself unusually sensitive to pollen, mold, or other allergic exposure, think about hidden food allergies contributing to your discomfort and consider the following advice.

Just knowing that this food allergy exists will often provide the clue that there is a reason for those days where your symptoms strike so severely. Your powers of observation should lead you to the foods or beverages you need to avoid.

Patients like Jim and Marlene are typical. I follow a general rule when I evaluate them:

◊ *Always think about hidden immediate food allergies in patients who react immediately to pollen, dust, or mold.*

This concept leads to a second general rule:

◊ *Treatment of severe immediate reactions should include reducing or eliminating minor food and environmental allergies so that major allergies can be better tolerated.*

In the case of hidden immediate food allergies, this concept means we should acknowledge these hidden food allergies and minimize their effect.

Minimizing Hidden Immediate Food Allergies

Minimizing the impact of hidden immediate food allergies sounds hard. Is it impossible? After all, many people who suffer quick-onset allergy symptoms react not to one food but to many. When we test these patients, many show hidden allergies to all the food we test. How can they avoid all these foods? They would have nothing left to eat.

Fortunately, minimizing these hidden food allergies is not as difficult as it sounds. To minimize your symptoms, use Mother Nature's forgetfulness. When she made hidden immediate food allergies, she forgot to give them a memory. This forgetfulness is to your advantage.

Rotate Your Diet

Most of these foods increase your symptoms only if you eat them daily. Eat them less often and they lose their power to torment you.

So rotate your foods so you do not eat them every day. Does this mean you have to sit down with pencil and paper and make a chart of all the food you will eat this week? Not at all!

Even sloppy rotation works. If you just avoid the habit of eating the same foods every day—for example, a peanut butter sandwich each noon—rotation will work.

What do you do with foods such as wheat and milk, which you might like to include in your diet daily? You can reduce the amount you eat or drink to the amount you tolerate without symptoms. A little experimenting with your diet should show you how much you tolerate. If you are sensitive to the MALS chemicals, reduce your consumption of the foods and beverages that contain them. Eating only this amount works well in keeping you comfortable and your allergy bucket uncrowded.

In the section "The Rotation Diet" in Chapter 6, I will show you how you can rotate your foods if you feel uncomfortable making a rotation up. Now we will spend time reviewing how you should respond to immediate food allergy symptoms.

Dealing with Your Immediate Food Allergy

We have already discussed how you should deal with these quickly appearing classic or MALS food allergy symptoms. Now is a good time to summarize the actions you can take to avoid these symptoms.

Your best treatment of immediate food allergy is to cast these offending foods out of your diet. If you neither eat nor drink them, they cannot bring you pain and discomfort. Often your elimination need not be complete; limiting the amount you consume to the amount you tolerate will keep you free of pain and/or discomfort.

Finding the Foods

Some of these foods are obvious. Avoiding the foods that cause your reactions works well when you know which foods to avoid. As we discussed, in the following syndromes the offending food sticks out like a strawberry in a bowl of oatmeal.

If you suffer anaphylaxis, the peanut that quickly chokes your breathing, the shrimp that swells your tongue, the MSG that cramps your intestines, or the strawberry that makes your skin break out in hives cannot hide. You know that the shrimp, peanut, MSG, or strawberry sparked your reaction.

The fresh fruits and vegetables that cause oral allergy syndrome typically leave no doubt in your mind. As your mouth swells and itches, you know that the apple or the carrot you are eating is guilty.

However, some of these foods are not obvious. In other conditions of immediate food allergies, the foods that trouble you are not so apparent. They hide their identity from you. You must find them because you cannot exclude them from your diet until you determine which foods cause your symptoms.

We saw that offending foods can mask themselves by causing symptoms hours after your meal. The exercise anaphylaxis that interrupts your jog or your exercise class is a good example. If you do not know about exercise anaphylaxis, you will not realize its genesis in immediate food allergy; you will not even suspect food. Even if you know about exercise anaphylaxis you are still left with a puzzle: Which food, among the many you ate before exercising, made you sick?

If you are unsure which foods caused your exercise reaction, you will need to find skilled help to diagnose your food allergy. Ask your doctor or other medical professional who cares for you to assist you in your search. If you cannot find help in diagnosing the foods that cause your reaction, review the suggestions in the chapter on exercise anaphylaxis. They suggest measures you can take to find the culprit foods and avoid scary reactions while you exercise.

If You React to One or a Few Foods

If you know which foods to avoid, your course of action is clear. Avoid them! If you do not know which foods make you ill, try an elimination diet. Stop eating the foods you suspect, especially those I have already mentioned in preceding sections. After avoiding these foods for a week, start eating them again, every day. If you tolerate eating them once a day, try eating them as part of two or more meals each day. Eating them frequently will reveal those foods that cause symptoms only when eaten in excess.

If you are allergic to one or a few foods, this approach should help you find them.

If You React to Many Foods

The problem of finding your culprit foods becomes more difficult when you react to many foods. As we discussed, people with hay fever, hives, and other immediate allergies often suffer from multiple food allergies caused by reactions to the proteins shared between pollen and foods.

Although you may not be able to identify these foods, you can deal with them. In most cases they cause mild symptoms; rotating your diet makes their symptoms even milder. Eating these foods for one, two, or three days and then avoiding them for the next day will often prevent your food reaction.

Multiple food allergies often cause you so little trouble that you notice them only when you are already reacting to another allergy, such as pollen hay fever. As we saw, many of my patients find that their sneezing, wheezing, or itching troubles them less if they rotate their diet in the spring when the tree and grass pollens fly, or in the fall when oppressive ragweed pollens take to the air.

If you are reacting against the protein in foods, consider rotating your diet when pollen or other allergens make you suffer. With MALS food allergy, reduce your intake of foods with excess food chemicals. These diet changes will not cure you, but they may make a miserable day a little less uncomfortable.

Emptying the Bucket

Dealing with your food allergies frequently involves more than restricting your diet. Reducing your exposure to pollen, dust mites, mold, or animal dander can give you surprisingly effective food allergy relief.

By correcting allergic exposures in your environment, you empty your bucket of the allergens you breathe. Now you have made more room in your bucket for your food allergies. You weaken their power to hurt you. With your bucket partially empty, you may find that you can eat a limited amount of the foods that would otherwise bring you pain and discomfort.

However, even if you reduce your pollen, dust mite, mold, or pet allergy, you will not be able to eat everything you desire. You still must somewhat limit your intake of the food or foods that bother you. However, you should be delighted with your less stringent diet while enjoying fewer headaches and less sneezing, itching, and hives.

Reducing the Impact of Dust Mite, Mold, Pollen, and Animal Dander

We should review here two actions you can take to reduce this impact, avoiding exposure and receiving treatment with allergy injections.

Avoiding Exposure

As the best treatment of food allergy is avoidance, the best treatment of dust mite, pollen, mold, and animal dander allergies is the same. Limit or eliminate your exposure, and you limit or eliminate your symptoms.

How to do this is too detailed to include in this book about food allergy. However, I would like to discuss one treatment of these non-food allergies that quiets food allergy, often putting it to sleep. It is a treatment that allergists use: allergy injections.

Allergy Injections

Again, I hesitate to explore allergy injections deeply, as you may have no opportunity to use this treatment. Or perhaps your medical caregiver uses other effective treatments in the place of allergy injection treatment. I mention this treatment only because this information may help you.

Allergy injections contain the same dust mite, pollen, mold, and animal dander that cause allergy symptoms such as sneezing, wheezing, and itching. We inject tiny amounts of dust mite, pollen, mold, and animal dander under the skin from once a week to once a month, depending on your stage of treatment. The injections lower sensitivity to these allergens by calming the immune system, curtailing its mistaken fight against harmless dust mite, mold, pollen, and animal dander. They dampen unpleasant symptoms such as sneezing, wheezing, and itching.

Why would we use this treatment if you could eliminate your symptoms by eliminating the exposures that cause them? Because you may not be able to eliminate them. Perhaps you live in a musty basement apartment or live over a musty basement at home and you cannot make it dry. Alternatively, you may work in a moldy building or attend a musty school. If you cannot move to another apartment or home, if you must attend the musty school or workplace, then you cannot avoid these exposures.

When medicines such as antihistamines and decongestants fail to quiet your symptoms from breathing these allergens, you can use allergy injections to lessen your discomfort from these unavoidable exposures. They can reduce the impact of both classic and MALS food allergies.

For years our patients have told me that allergy injections to dust mite, mold, pollen, and animal dander lessen their food allergy symptoms. With treatment, our patients can eat foods that, before treatment, they had to avoid. We discussed part of the reason why injections help: by relieving these environmental allergies, they reduce our patient's allergic load. They partially empty their allergy bucket. Our patient's ability to eat foods rises, while food-bred distress relents.

In addition, scientific studies show a further—and curious—effect of allergy injections: they directly reduce allergy to food directed against the proteins of foods.

We saw that foods share many of the proteins of pollen that cause hay fever. In addition to the pollen/food relations we discussed, there are indications that house dust mite shares protein allergens with crustaceans and snails. After all, Mother Nature likes to use the same proteins in different plants.

These shared proteins are especially pertinent if you suffer from the oral allergy syndrome. As you receive allergy injections of pollen protein, the injections quiet not only your reaction to pollen protein but also your reactions to food protein that make your mouth swell with the oral allergy syndrome. They can similarly help quiet other protein-directed food allergies.

When allergy injections aren't possible. For various reasons, including inability to afford this treatment or lack of a doctor skilled in allergy injections, patients with food allergy may be unable to receive allergy injections. Much research now focuses on alternative treatments for these people, including administering dust mite, pollen, and mold antigens by mouth, or injecting substances that halt the allergic reaction. Check for the availability of this care with your medical caregiver.

When to Visit an Allergist

If your food allergy is mild and the culprit foods apparent, you should be able to treat yourself. Follow the suggestions that we discussed. If you suffer greatly and you do not know the cause of your suffering, you should consult your primary health care professional.

Should this health care professional be an allergist? Not necessarily. Other medical care professionals may offer you significant help; allergy injections may not be the only treatment option open to you. Discuss your symptoms with your primary caregiver—many understand allergy and will help you find the foods that trouble you. She or he may be able to guide you to a diet that minimizes your symptoms. Only when your caregiver suggests that you seek allergy care should you consult an allergist.

Immediate or quick-reacting symptoms are not the only symptoms caused by allergy to food. Delayed symptoms also cause much pain and discomfort, a subject we will now explore.

Delayed Food Symptoms in Classic and MALS Food Allergy

Unlike rapidly striking immediate food symptoms, delayed food symptoms move like slugs. Hours, a day, or more time passes before these slowpokes stir to action. Because they move so slowly, they confuse doctors and breed misinformation, misinformation that even affects our allergy literature.

Many medical articles tell us that few people react to food. This is not true—researchers miss their patients' food allergy because the researchers pay too much attention to symptoms that strike quickly after eating. They tend to ignore those that start slowly. If they would only look for these delayed food symptoms, they would find that they commonly affect their patients.

Delayed food symptoms occur at least as frequently as immediate food symptoms among my patients. I suspect that such symptoms are even more common; my patients tell me that they suffer many symptoms that start hours after they eat.

Those suffering delayed food reactions suffer many of the same symptoms that bother those suffering immediate food reactions. These symptoms are the same whether their genesis arises from classic food allergy or from MALS food allergies.

Either immediate or delayed symptoms make your head hurt, your intestines cramp, your skin itch, or your tongue swell. Either stuffs up your nose, gives you a choking feeling in your air passages, or makes you wheeze. They differ in how quickly symptoms appear after a meal. No part of your body can hide from the pain and discomfort of the immediate or delayed food reactions from either classic or MALS food allergies.

The cause arising from both MALS and classic food allergies and the delay between eating and suffering confuse not only researchers and doctors, but also the people who suffer delayed allergy symptoms. Why would they think that yesterday's corn on the cob caused today's stuffy nose? Would they realize that last night's wheat cereal makes them feel groggy, tired, and unable to concentrate this morning? That the sweet roll they ate yesterday afternoon contributes to this morning's headaches? When they fail to connect the food they ate yesterday with the misery they suffer today, they cannot remove from their diets the foods that make them sick.

If you understand how delayed food symptoms act, you can learn if you suffer from these symptoms. To help you reach this understanding, let's review the characteristics of delayed symptoms and examine how they differ from immediate symptoms.

Characteristics of Delayed Food Symptoms

They need a large amount of food to trigger them. Not only do they start slowly, they also won't start until you eat large quantities of food, much more than the tiny amount of food that sparks immediate symptoms such as for anaphylaxis. You must also eat more than the tiny amount that makes the mouth and the throat swell with hives in the oral allergy syndrome.

They often travel in a group. MALS food allergy typically arises from a group of foods containing excess chemicals. Although immediate classic food reactions usually involve one or a few foods, delayed classic food symptoms can involve many foods, all at the same time. We see this pattern on our skin tests. Many of our patients show allergy to the proteins of two, four, or a dozen foods. Some even show allergies to every food tested, a condition I call "global" food allergy. Needless to say, this diagnosis surprises them.

"I reacted to all the foods on the skin test. Do you mean I cannot eat anything? I can't live without eating!" many tell me with great distress. My answer is always the same: "It's not that bad; you can eat all these foods, but you must use some caution."

They are very easy to miss. Delayed food symptoms confuse doctors and patients because they start slowly, need large feedings, and often involve many foods. Patients typically ask questions such as: "Surely I can't react to something I ate last night?" They also ask, "Can I be allergic to wheat if I can eat it at times without trouble?" Or, "I can't be allergic to three foods at once, can I?"

The answer to all three questions is yes.

If you think that these delayed food symptoms sound like the deeply hidden immediate food symptoms we discussed, you are right. They are opposite side of the same coin. Their main difference is the speed at which they bring illness.

Both immediate and delayed symptoms may operate at the same time. My patients with food allergies often react both right away and hours later.

For instance, Karen knows that popcorn makes her nose stuff up while she eats it—an immediate symptom. It also makes her stomach churn and ache many hours later—a delayed symptom. This combination is no surprise. Many scientific studies show that the same allergen can cause both immediate and delayed symptoms. Not only do foods act this way, so do allergies to dust mite, mold, and pollen.

Sometimes there are only delayed symptoms. Not all of my patients show the immediate symptoms of food allergy—they suffer no sneezing, wheezing, or itching right after they eat. Since they show no immediate reaction to tip off the diagnosis, their medical care providers can overlook food allergy. So you do not make this mistake, you need to be aware of this often sneaky illness.

Once you learn about delayed food allergy symptoms, you can fight its ability to confuse you. If you understand delayed food allergy's slowness to react, ability to involve multiple foods, and dependence on adequate intake of culprit foods, you can search for the foods that cause your delayed symptoms.

If you eat a food infrequently—once a week to once a month—you should notice if this food causes you pain and discomfort. For instance, you should notice if you suffer a headache, whether immediate or delayed, after your twice-monthly feast of popcorn at the movies. However, you will find it more difficult to identify an offending food if you eat it frequently—daily or several times a week. Then your symptoms will be with you daily, not seeming to be caused by your diet. Three foods fit in this category—milk, wheat, and corn. Because they are so important in your diet, and because each food can cause varying illnesses, we will cover them in some detail in the following chapter.

CHAPTER 5

Foods That Are Common in Our Diet and Present Unusual Problems

Milk

I knew I had to tell you about the illnesses caused by milk.

I was the guest on a radio talk show, and the hour was speeding along nicely. Calls poured in from listeners with questions about their allergies, and as usual, the callers' questions were astute and insightful. I was doing what I love to do—tell my patients' stories to people who can learn from them.

One of our callers was Kathy, and our conversation went like this: "Dr. Walsh, I want to tell you about my allergy.

"I used to have a terribly stuffed-up nose," she said. "It was so stuffy that it blocked off completely at night and I had to breathe through my mouth. All this mouth breathing made my mouth so dry that it woke me up at night. Many mornings I felt like I hadn't slept.

"I went to an allergist, who did skin tests and told me that my stuffy nose was not caused by an allergy. When I asked him if drinking milk could cause my stuffy nose, he said, 'No, it couldn't.'

"I asked my chiropractor the same question, and he thought it was a good possibility. He suggested that I stop drinking milk for a week and see what happened. I stopped, and my nose cleared up; I can breathe through it. I sleep well at night—no dry mouth, and I feel better than I have felt in years."

Kathy suffered for years—and suffered unnecessarily. Her sensitivity to milk brought uncomfortable nasal stuffiness to her days and troubled sleep to her nights. If she had only known about milk reactions, she would have responded appropriately and spared herself years of breathing through a nose that felt like it was blocked with mud. She should never have heard an allergist say that milk could not cause her suffering. It can, and it did.

Her story convinced me that I must write about milk. Many people suffer from drinking milk, and they need to know why they suffer.

Before telling you about how milk causes illnesses, let me acknowledge its benefits:

◇ Without milk, survival of the young would be difficult.
◇ Milk contains all the food elements needed for growth and good health.
◇ Milk is the leading source of calcium and a good source of phosphorus.
◇ No food has gained greater acceptability or offers a greater variety of uses than milk.

However, we must now look at its defects, specifically its ability to cause milk-sensitive people to suffer.

Milk can trouble you in three ways:

◇ You be allergic to milk.
◇ Milk can cause milk/mucus blockage.
◇ You may have lactose intolerance—the inability to digest milk sugar.

Milk causes a variety of other reactions, some very rare. We will not discuss these rare reactions but will concentrate on the common but often unappreciated ways in which milk troubles people.

You May Be Allergic to Milk

Milk can cause both immediate and delayed allergic symptoms. For the milk-allergic person, it can ignite any of the many illnesses of food allergy. Milk makes Mary's head ache and her son Matt's stomach hurt.

It makes Charlotte sneeze and Jim break out in hives. It brings on Dee's terrible tiredness and Chuck's irritability. Milk causes these allergic symptoms and many more.

Immediate allergy to milk. For people who react within minutes of drinking milk, symptoms strike quickly and usually after drinking even a small amount. If you react quickly to milk, even a small swallow of milk may cause you great distress.

Like all immediate reactions, they usually surprise you and can even scare you. If you drink milk and suddenly find your skin welting and itching, your stomach hurting, or your chest tightening, you have every right to be surprised and even scared. Typically, these symptoms appear so dramatically, you know you are allergic to milk.

Delayed allergy to milk. Delayed reactions to milk can appear hours after you drink it. Like all delayed reactions, it moves slowly. With this delay, milk-allergic people can easily overlook the cause. Further obscuring the cause, they react only when they drink too much milk; smaller quantities are tolerated well.

If you suffer delayed reactions to milk, you may miss its contribution to your pain and discomfort, as you could miss any delayed allergy. You may fail to tie together these "flu" symptoms with milk because they may not appear every time you drink it, but only when you drink more than you can tolerate.

Milk Can Cause Milk/Mucus Blockage

Immediate and delayed reactions to milk are not the only ways by which milk can bother you. It can block your breathing, a blockage I call milk/mucus blockage. I believe that this blockage bothers my call-in questioner Kathy.

Symptoms. In many people, milk sets off an oppressive outpouring of mucus from the nose and sinuses. This mucus fills the nose and pours down the throat. If you are affected, this heavy mucus can make your stomach hurt and nauseate you.

Mucus also can well up in the airways leading to your lungs—the tracheal and the bronchial air passages. A feeling of itching or a lump in your throat may accompany the mucus, forcing a maddening cough as you fruitlessly try to relieve this irritation. Often this cough is loud and persistent, frequently coming in jackhammerlike spasms, frustrating not only you but also those who are near you and hear you. If your child is affected, you may wonder if he or she has pneumonia; if your spouse is affected, you may banish him or her to another bed so you can sleep.

If this sounds familiar to you, rest assured it sounds familiar to many others as well. Many of my patients come to me for treatment knowing that milk blocks their noses and makes them blow out and cough up mucus. However, others come unaware that this healthful beverage causes their annoying nose blockage.

Milk/mucus blockage rarely shows up on skin tests. Milk is not the only cause of this very common allergic cough. Many foods and environmental exposures also provoke the cough, so many that neither the patient nor I may think of milk allergy when we look for the cause. It would be nice if our milk skin tests would remind us of this possibility, but the skin test almost never shows milk allergy. Either it cannot detect this type of milk allergy, or allergy does not cause the milk/mucus blockage.

I believe that the reason why milk skin tests fail to help us is that milk/mucus blockage is not an allergic reaction. Instead, I visualize it as a defect in my patients' ability to digest some protein or fat of milk.

Perhaps people affected by milk/mucus blockage lack an enzyme necessary for digestion. When they drink milk their bodies don't like it, can't handle it, and eliminate it by dumping it into the nose and the air passages of the lungs. Then, coughing and nose-blowing flush the milk fat or protein out of the body the same way we flush a toilet. This thought may not be too far-fetched. Milk is unusual in that it contains more fatty acids and derivatives (components of fat) than any other food—about five hundred. Many enter the body from the intestines unchanged and travel to the liver for digestion.

If the liver cannot digest them, the body may be forced to dispose of them through the nose and airways, just as we dispose of our garbage in a trash can. Then the nasal and airway mucus hauls them away, prompting the stuffiness, wheezing, and heavy mucus production many of us suffer.

Milk's proteins are similar to its fats—many are found only in milk. If the body cannot digest these proteins, it may similarly dispose of them in the nose and air passages.

You May Have Lactose Intolerance— the Inability to Digest Milk Sugar

In our diet, milk is unique. Not only does it contain fats and proteins found in no other food, it also contains a sugar—lactose—found in no other food. In many people this special sugar causes illness.

Lactose is a complex sugar made up of two simple sugars harnessed together like two racehorses hitched head-to-head. The horses cannot enter the race until someone frees them from each other. Similarly, the simple sugars of lactose cannot enter the bloodstream from the intestines (be absorbed) while they are hitched together. As long as they are joined, they must remain in the intestine.

They can only race into the body after they are freed from each other in the intestine. An enzyme in the intestine, lactase, frees them.

Lactose intolerance in the newborn. When infants are born with too little lactase to split these sugars, their health is compromised and their existence threatened. The lactose trapped in the intestine causes acid diarrhea, and the baby is unable to digest food.

Fortunately, family doctors and pediatricians know this threatening illness well and, under their care, lactose is removed from the infants' diet and replaced with soy or other formula. They survive, and they grow robustly. However, in the adult, lactose intolerance is often undiagnosed, although it is frequently present.

Lactose intolerance in the adult. Mother Nature designed milk to be food for infants. Never dreaming that we would drink milk beyond the baby years, she invested little effort in creating the lactase-production system.

Although some people digest milk sugar without harm all their lives, others lose that ability as they mature into children and adults. As their lactase-producing system ages, they fail to make enough lactase to split lactose's simple sugars. The intact lactose molecule cannot enter the body; it remains trapped in the intestine.

Further showing her indifference to the lactase-producing system, Mother Nature placed it on the surface of the intestine, where it is easily injured. Viral diarrheas such as stomach flu strip it away. That's why many doctors ask their patients with viral diarrheas to reduce their consumption of milk. Although the lactase production eventually recovers to preinfection levels, for a while the person recovering from a viral gastroenteritis can experience lactose intolerance.

Who is susceptible to lactose intolerance? Some people are more susceptible to lactase deficiency—lactose intolerance—than others. In general, people from nondairying parts of the world lose their lactase enzyme easily; as milk has not been a traditional part of their diet, they seem to have lost their ability to digest milk. Seventy percent of people of African, Asian, Middle Eastern, Mediterranean, and Native American ancestry experience decline in their lactose digestion ability. In contrast, only about 5 percent of people with northern European ancestors and 15 percent of those with central European forebears whose traditional diet included milk suffer diminished lactase ability.

How lactose causes symptoms. Why does it matter that people with lactose intolerance cannot absorb lactose? Because the unabsorbed lactose trapped in the intestine sops up water like a sponge, drawing large amounts of water into the intestine.

Filled with water, the intestine gurgles and cramps, pushing this water to our colon and rectum until we finally expel it all into the toilet in a watery diarrhea. Because sugar is acid, the diarrhea is acid, and it often burns the rectal area.

To make matters worse, although we cannot digest lactose, many of the germs that live in our intestine can and are only too happy to do so. As they greedily eat the lactose, they release gas that adds to the gurgling and cramping as the water-lactose-gas makes its tortuous way through our hurting intestine. The crowning insult from these germs is the sewer-gas fragrance these gases release (politely referred to as flatulence) to embarrass the poor lactose intolerance sufferer.

If lactose-digesting ability is only diminished, not completely absent, symptoms are much milder. There may be only mild cramping or excess gas as signs of this diminished ability.

There are two further points you need to know about milk sensitivity. First, symptoms caused by milk and cheese, although they seem to arise from the same allergies, can have entirely different causes. If you do not understand the differences, you can be easily confused. Second, we will discuss the most important information you should know—if you are sensitive to milk.

Milk and Cheese Allergy

In the previous section we looked at sensitivity to milk; drinking milk can cause you pain and discomfort. You can also suffer similar symptoms from eating cheese, but the cause may be entirely different. You must understand this difference in causes because it will show you how classic and MALS food allergies can be confused.

Reactions to Milk and Cheese Can Have Entirely Different Causes

If you react to cheese, your reaction may not be caused by an allergy to the milk protein from which the cheese is made. "Whoa," you say, "that can't be right! After all, isn't cheese made from milk?"

Yes, it is.

"Then aren't milk allergy and cheese allergy really the same?"

Not always.

In making cheese, the cheesemaker concentrates the protein of milk and then mixes it with cultures of special bacteria that process the milk protein into cheese. Now, milk protein is a large molecule made up of amino acids chained together like the links in the chain of a necklace.

If you needed to take apart a necklace, you would unhook one link in the chain from another. Soon you would be left with a pile of individual necklace links—you had separated the necklace into its component parts. The bacteria in the cheese culture operate on milk protein like you operated on the necklace: they take apart the milk protein by unhooking one amino acid from another—fermentation—when they change milk protein into cheese. The longer the cheese is fermented, the more time they have to separate the milk proteins into amino acids.

Why does that matter? It matters because a troublesome amino acid makes up a large part of the protein of milk. This amino acid is called glutamic acid. Once freed from milk protein, it is called MSG or monosodium glutamate. This amino acid is one of the causes of MALS food allergy, bringing many people great distress.

Cheese contains MSG. To restate the problem, making cheese frees large amounts of glutamic acid from milk protein, making cheese a food containing a large quantity of free glutamic acid or MSG. The longer cheese is fermented, the more time bacteria have to free glutamic acid from milk protein, and the more free MSG the cheese contains.

Therefore, if you know that eating cheese makes your head throb, your stomach cramp, or your breathing wheeze, you may think that milk protein allergy causes your distress. You might say you suffer from classic food allergy directed against milk protein.

You could be mistaken; the MSG in the cheese may be causing your symptoms. You may needlessly avoid milk, which does not hurt you, and continue to use foods containing MSG, which do.

Other cultured foods with MSG. Milk protein cultured with bacteria makes other foods in addition to cheese, and these foods also contain appreciable quantities of MSG. These foods include acidophilus milk, cultured buttermilk, sour cream, and yogurt, and each may contain enough MSG to bother MSG-sensitive people. If you share this sensitivity, your reaction to these foods may be caused by their MSG content, not by their milk protein content.

Other milk-derived foods also contain some levels of MSG. They include caseinates (made from the casein protein of milk) and hydrolyzed whey (the protein-rich watery part of milk separated from the curd and then hydrolyzed, or broken into amino acids). In both products, glutamic acid has been freed from protein and changed to MSG, in these cases by an operation called acid-base processing. Again, MSG-sensitive people may not be reacting to milk if they suffer after eating these foods.

Now you should not be confused about the difference between milk and cheese allergy. Cheese and other high-MSG foods can make you sick, either because of MALS food allergy or because you suffer classic allergy to milk protein. Sometimes both allergies operate together.

Having examined the ways milk can make you ill, let us proceed to the topic so important to you: how you can determine if you are sensitive to milk and how to respond to this allergy.

Identifying and Treating Your Milk Reaction

We have looked at the three ways in which milk can bother you: you may be allergic to milk; you may suffer from milk/mucus blockage; or you may have lactose intolerance—the inability to digest milk sugar.

Now we need to examine the steps you take to determine if you suffer from any of these three milk reactions. We can list these steps as follows:

◊ You must notice your sensitivity.
◊ Take milk out of your diet for a week and then return it to your diet.

Each of these steps is simple, but many people continue to suffer because they do not take them. Make sure you do not make this mistake.

You Must Notice Your Sensitivity

If milk bothers you, you need to notice that you are bothered. Seems obvious, doesn't it? We have already discussed the importance of noticing your allergies. Unfortunately, many people who suffer from milk do not suspect it, and they cannot be helped until they notice this sensitivity. Do not be like them; think of milk sensitivity. It may be causing some of your symptoms.

Do you suffer abdominal discomfort or cramping pain? Does your stomach bloat? Does excessive gas embarrass you, or do you experience watery diarrhea? You may suffer from lactose intolerance—you may not be able to digest the lactose sugar in milk.

Do you suffer from a stuffy nose with lots of heavy mucus drainage? Perhaps you cough up copious amounts of mucus, with an annoying, persistent cough that exasperates your friends and irritates your loved ones. If you do, you may suffer from milk/mucus blockage.

Perhaps you are allergic to milk. This opens you to the plethora of symptoms that allergy brings to those it plagues—symptoms varying from the very apparent immediate reactions to flulike delayed symptoms. Headaches, body aches, stomach pains, and tiredness may be your gifts from that healthful drink of milk.

Take Milk out of Your Diet for a Week and Then Return It to Your Diet

If you suffer from milk in any of these ways, you can discover if milk causes your distress. It's simple. Take milk and other dairy products out of your diet for a week and see if your symptoms subside. Return them to your diet and see if your distress returns. If this trial period leaves you unsure, redo the test.

It works! You can diagnose your own milk sensitivity, whether it be allergy, milk/mucus blockage, or lactose intolerance.

Foods to Eliminate

Which foods do you eliminate during your milk-free trial? All forms of milk, such as whole milk, skim milk, and evaporated milk, as well as foods made from milk, such as ice cream and cheese. Butter is okay; it is composed of milk fat, not the protein that causes food protein allergy or the milk sugar that causes lactose intolerance.

Read the labels on the foods and drugs you use. Avoid any that contain lactose or that mention milk-derived ingredients such as foods made with casein or whey, both milk proteins.

Limit Your Milk Intake to the Amount You Tolerate

If you react quickly and violently to milk, you must completely avoid it. Your violent symptoms show that you suffer immediate allergy to milk, and drinking it may place you in danger of anaphylaxis.

If you are mildly sensitive. For many milk-sensitive people, complete avoidance is unnecessary. Many people with milk allergy, lactose intolerance, or milk/mucus blockage tolerate small amounts of milk with no troubling symptoms. They should use it in the small amounts they tolerate, because milk is an excellent food. For those suffering from lactose intolerance, lactase enzyme added to milk will reduce lactose to easily absorbable simple sugars. You also can buy milk already treated to remove some or all of the lactose. Either the enzyme preparation or the pretreated milk may let you drink milk without unpleasant consequences.

After an intestinal virus infection. Sometimes lactose intolerance (lactase deficiency) happens for a limited time after a virus intestinal infection such as a stomach flu. If so, for a limited period you may have to avoid milk, use a low-lactose milk, or add lactase to your milk. After your intestine recovers from the viral infection, you can return to using whole milk freely.

Yogurt and lactose. Yogurt contains the lactose of milk, but for lactose-intolerant people, it may be acceptable if it contains a live culture of bacteria. This live culture should be specified on the label.

In the stomach, bacteria from the live cultures split the lactose sugar into digestible simple sugars. However, they also continue the work of the bacteria that made the yogurt, further splitting protein into glutamic acid-rich amino acids, possibly bothering the MSG-sensitive person.

If you suffer MSG-caused symptoms, remember that yogurt contains some free MSG. It can cause you great discomfort, especially if added to other foods in your diet that also contain an elevated MSG content.

Irritable bowel and yogurt. This caution is especially pertinent for my patients with irritable bowel syndrome. Many of them experience increased abdominal symptoms when they eat too much MSG. When lactase deficiency is added to irritable bowel, they more readily suffer bloating, abdominal discomfort, diarrhea, and tiredness.

A caution. If you must restrict or eliminate milk, it seems wise to supplement your diet with calcium. Ask your medical caregiver for advice about calcium.

Milk Allergy in the Infant and the Young Child

For infants and young children, milk sensitivity is no simple problem because milk forms such an important part of their diet. What other food provides such nutrition or so much calcium for growing bones? How do you feed these young people?

The American Academy of Pediatrics has good advice. It estimates that milk allergy is rare, with only one child in a hundred truly allergic to cow's milk. If you suspect it, consult your primary caregiver before undertaking any corrective measures. Seek emergency help if your baby develops breathing difficulty, turns blue, looks pale or weak, swells in the head and neck area, or has bloody diarrhea.

It helps to breast-feed your baby for as long as possible, as studies indicate that fewer breast-fed babies develop milk allergy. This is an especially valuable precaution if anyone in the immediate family is allergy-prone. Introduce new foods to your baby's diet gradually, one every one to two weeks, while watching for signs of allergy.

The *Foods and Nutrition Encyclopedia* states the options succinctly:

◇ Substitute goat's milk. [Goat's milk will not end your symptoms if you are reacting to a protein found in both cow's milk and goat's milk. If so, eliminate both from your diet.]

◇ Change the form of the milk; that is, try boiled, powered, acidulated, or evaporated milk. [Sometimes processing the milk as mentioned above alters the protein that causes milk allergy, destroying its ability to cause illness. However, if the offending protein resists alteration by the above processes, this approach will not work.]

◇ Eliminate cow's milk and milk products from the diet, and substitute formulas in which the protein is derived from meat or soybeans.

The last option is usually chosen and usually is effective. However, if you choose a soybean formula, be aware that many infants and young children allergic to cow's milk protein also react to soy protein. Formulas where protein is hydrolyzed (broken into its constituent amino acids) should provide good nutrition and calcium.

Although hydrolyzed formula contains large amounts of free glutamic acid, your child may tolerate it well. Children seem to react less severely to the MALS chemicals than adults do. However, be careful if you or another member of your family reacts to MSG; your infant may show this sensitivity by wheezing, crying with colic, or other symptoms. Watch for these symptoms if you use a hydrolyzed formula.

Be sure to consult with your medical professional before making any formula changes.

Milk Allergy in the Adult

For adults who cannot tolerate any milk, eliminating it from the diet relieves their symptoms—no more milk, no more suffering. For those adults who tolerate small amounts of milk, limiting their diets to this small amount similarly relieves milk-caused symptoms.

Milk Sensitivity in My Practice

As I was writing about milk, I wondered about how many of my patients suffer from it. To answer this question, one day I asked each of the patients I saw if milk bothered them. Many said it did; if they drank too much milk, they suffered stuffy noses, wheezing, abdominal distress, or other symptoms. They knew they must restrict its use or eliminate it. Most had discovered this before coming to see me, alerted to the possibility by their primary-care doctor, another medical caregiver, a family member, a friend, or by their own good observation.

I believe that the patients I questioned that day limit their milk intake because milk troubles them. As this number includes more than half of the adults I questioned, the conclusion is plain: milk sensitivity affects many allergic patients.

Some examples: Bernie and Joan told me that young Travis coughs until he vomits when he drinks milk. Gayle suffers both low and high back pain when she drinks milk. She also suffers bloating all over her body, most noticeable on the face. Painful cramps march through her intestine, and she feels tired and cold.

Cathy suffers the same bloating and draining tiredness from drinking milk. In addition, her nose stuffs up and terrible migraine headaches strike.

My experience convinces me that milk sensitivity bothers many of my patients. Many cannot drink it without suffering a variety of distressing symptoms, including cough, congestion, bloating, back pain, and terrible tiredness.

Many of my patients suffer from milk in more than one way. For instance, they may suffer symptoms of milk allergy plus lactose intolerance or milk/mucus blockage. In addition, many suffer MALS allergy to the MSG in milk-derived food products. If you discover that milk makes you suffer from one of these illnesses, look also for the others.

Please understand milk sensitivity; it may affect you or a loved one who needs your help. Above all, do not allow yourself to suffer from milk because you have not noticed how it hurts you.

Wheat

Allergy to wheat is a good example of an allergic reaction caused by classic food allergy—the protein of food. Wheat does not contain high quantities of the MALS chemicals—sugar, citrus, MSG or low-calorie sweeteners—unless the baker introduced these chemicals during manufacture of a wheat-based food.

Without doubt, wheat is the foundation of our modern diet. It makes our daily breads, crackers, rolls, and breakfast cereals. It thickens our soups and puddings, it makes our pasta. Remove wheat, and our diets shrink unpleasantly.

Unfortunately, people with wheat allergy must either eat less wheat or eat none—their diet is truly restricted and austere. I discovered how restrictive years ago from a patient's father. When I asked Jim how his son was doing, he replied, "He's doing all right as long as he doesn't eat wheat. He wheezes badly if he eats it."

Jim then described the difficulty of providing an adequate diet for his son while avoiding wheat. He purchases wheat substitutes at natural health food stores and co-ops; we will discuss these food substitutes. His wife bakes special wheat-free breads, crackers, and other foods. Although the diet helps his son, to make it work Jim must use intelligence and determination.

Wheat allergy can limit the diet severely or affect it hardly at all. Two factors determine the degree of limitation: how quickly symptoms strike and how hard they strike.

Quickly Striking Wheat Allergy Symptoms

We already discussed immediate allergy to foods, with the quick-striking anaphylaxis being a good example. In susceptible people eating wheat can trip off anaphylaxis that appears quickly as they eat it, or hours later when they exercise.

Wheat anaphylaxis acts the same as anaphylaxis to peanut, shrimp, or other foods. Sneezing, wheezing, hives, breathing blockage, and/or plunging blood pressure may strike abruptly. These dangerous reactions can frighten you, and you should be frightened; after eating wheat, some people have died.

Now, after making that frightening statement, let me be reassuring. Death caused by wheat is exceedingly rare; I can't remember the last time I saw a patient with a threatening wheat reaction. Wheat seldom causes these severe reactions, and when they occur, the symptoms usually act more like characters in a Halloween spook house, more frightening than dangerous.

Slowly Developing Wheat Allergy Symptoms

Symptoms that develop hours to days after eating wheat—delayed food symptoms—lack the dangerous punch of the quickly striking wheat reactions. You do not experience the fearsome gasping for breath or plummeting blood pressure.

Instead, delayed wheat allergy symptoms resemble other delayed food allergies—they bring annoying pain and discomfort, like the symptoms caused by virus infections such as the flu. You feel tired and achy, your stomach hurts, or your head throbs. Your thinking slows—my patients call it "spacey thinking."

At first you are sure you suffer from the flu, but your symptoms do not relent in a week or two, as you would expect with the flu. As you continue to experience pain and discomfort week after week and then month after month, you start to think that a delayed food reaction may be causing your discomfort.

We discussed how delayed food allergy, including the allergy caused by wheat, often hides its villainous activity from the people it torments. Because its symptoms occur hours after eating, they may not suspect it.

Delayed symptoms caused by wheat further confuse by appearing and disappearing without explanation—there is no law mandating that wheat must cause symptoms every time it is eaten. One week you are tired and irritable, and you can't breathe well. Your head throbs, your muscles and joints hurt, your stomach aches, and you suffer diarrhea. The next week you feel fine.

You may not realize that you suffer from wheat allergy; you may instead suspect chronic fatigue-headache syndrome or fibromyalgia. Actually, all of your suspicions may be right: all three illnesses can affect you at the same time.

Chronic Fatigue-Headache Syndrome: Leah's Story

I was not aware of delayed wheat allergy's power to disrupt lives until Leah brought it forcibly to my attention. I had treated her for years, trying to stop her chronic and painful headaches. I also tried to ease the great tiredness she suffered. In spite of all of my treatments, she still suffered distressing pain that at times was disabling.

Happily, all that changed! One day Leah told me that her headaches had stopped. Delighted, I asked her what happened.

"I stopped eating wheat," she replied. "After several days my headaches and tiredness disappeared, and I feel better than I have felt in years."

Leah's story surprised me because I had never suspected that wheat was responsible for some of her tiredness and headaches. I suspected dust mites, mold, and pollen, which cause headaches in many of my patients. I also suspected MALS food allergy, which does the same.

To a degree, I was right. All of these allergies bother Leah; she must be cautious about what she eats, and she must avoid the allergens in her home and workplace. In addition, to feel well she must also avoid wheat. Even a small amount brings debilitating headaches and tiredness.

I complemented Leah on her keen powers of observation. I also learned from her experience. Since she taught me about this wheat reaction, I have seen it in other patients, who owe the improvement in their brightness and concentration not to me but to her.

I wonder how many other people unknowingly suffer tiredness and headache from sensitivity to wheat.

Mild Wheat Allergy

Mild allergy to wheat is common. We see it frequently in our patients, signaled by a small wheat reaction on skin tests. Eating wheat seems to cause either no symptoms or only mild symptoms if too much is eaten. If symptoms bother the patient, mild reduction of wheat intake is all that is needed.

Moderate Wheat Allergy

Many wheat allergy sufferers react more strongly to wheat. They often show larger positive skin test reactions when we test wheat. Although they do not need to avoid it completely, they must be more cautious about how much wheat they eat each day.

Sometimes environmental conditions make mild wheat reactions more troublesome than they need be. This happens when patients' exposure to dust, mold, and/or animals is especially high in a musty house or apartment. These large exposures produce a state of heightened allergy, "priming" patients to suffer increased food allergy symptoms, even to foods that should cause only mild or no distress. Wheat-sensitive patients who live with excess mite, mold, or animal dander often find they can eat little wheat.

Some measures a person with moderate wheat sensitivity can take include:

◇ moderating wheat consumption
◇ rotating wheat with other grains
◇ combating the heightened reactivity to pollen, dust, mold, and animal dander with appropriate environmental corrections

Severe Wheat Allergy

Quick-striking symptoms belong here. People suffering these severe symptoms usually know that wheat caused them and that they must avoid wheat. I seldom find wheat to be a cause of delayed exercise anaphylaxis.

Some people with late-developing symptoms such as chronic fatigue and headaches have strong allergy to wheat and must eliminate it from their diet. The late development of symptoms sometimes confuses the diagnosis. If delayed wheat allergy is suspected, avoiding wheat for a week and then eating lots of wheat the next week should confirm the diagnosis.

A Case Study

I know Jamie well after years of treating her for wheezing and hay fever.

"I still have to be so careful of the foods I eat, Dr. Walsh," she said.

"It took years for me to give up sugar and diet pop, and I still miss them. If I drink a diet pop my throat itches and I develop a hacking cough. Too many acidic foods such as pasta sauce or tomatoes bring on a severely painful headache. Unfortunately, that means I cannot eat many of the foods I enjoy so much!"

Another illness, not caused by allergy, also restricts Jamie's choice of foods. This illness further complicates her diet and forces her to avoid other foods that make up a large part of our modern diet. Knowing about these further restrictions, I wondered about her allergy to corn and wheat and asked her if they still bothered her.

"Yes, they do, Dr. Walsh. Like acidic foods, wheat and corn bring on severe headaches. I can eat a little corn but not much or my head hurts. Because my diet is so restricted, it's hard to avoid eating bread. I love whole wheat bread, but I suffer if I eat it. I eat only white bread, as it seems to hurt me less."

Jamie had one extra revelation that reminded me of stories told to me by other patients. After eating a potato or a pizza, sleepiness descends on her as if she hadn't slept for days. She said with a wry chuckle, "I once went to a meeting soon after eating a baked potato. I no sooner sat down than I fell sound asleep. I felt so embarrassed."

Because of the success of my previous food allergy books, we see many people with complicated food allergies, often from states far from Minnesota. Many share Jamie's food restrictions. Like Jamie, their diet is so limited that only they can understand it. Only they know how to follow it. With all my experience in food allergy, how they achieve a balanced diet baffles me. Nevertheless, they learn to follow these diets, each in her or his own innovative way. To Jamie and to our other patients similarly affected, good for you. You are ingenious!

Another type of strong wheat allergy exists, a type so troublesome that we need to examine it separately. It is called celiac disease, and we will look at it in the next section. Of all of the food allergies I treat, it worries me the most.

Gluten Intolerance and Wheat Allergy

Wheat allergy truly worries me. To help you understand this worry, let's look at wheat in more detail.

Wheat is a complex food made of many components. One component, gluten, deserves our attention. We use it widely in our diet; we eat it every day. Unfortunately, some of us react adversely to gluten and may not realize its role in our illness.

What Is Gluten?

Gluten is the name of a variety of proteins found in wheat. These proteins possess an unusual ability—they glue foods together. Bakers and homemakers know this gluing activity so well that the word "glue" itself is derived from the word "gluten."

This gluing ability of gluten gives bread both elasticity and strength. The elasticity of gluten helps to trap carbon dioxide in the bread dough while the baker kneads it, forming the air bubbles that give bread its fluffiness. The strength of gluten holds the bread of your sandwich together as you eat it; without gluten, the bread would crumble into your lap.

Because it thickens and binds food products, bakers use gluten to make many food products, including breakfast cereal, crackers, soups, sauces, desserts, and snack foods. Because so many food products contain it, you buy it in many manufactured food products. If you are sensitive to gluten you must read the label of every food you purchase to avoid it.

Sources of Gluten

Wheat is not the only source of gluten. Rye, oats, and barley also contain gluten, and these grains can cause serious illness in gluten-sensitive people. They must avoid rye, oats, and barley and use substitute foods. (There is some evidence that the level of gluten is low in oats, and some oats may be acceptable in a gluten-free diet.)

Fortunately, substitutes exist. Flours made from corn and rice can substitute for flour from grain. Flours from starchy vegetables such as potatoes, or from legumes such as soybeans and lima beans, also provide acceptable substitutes. These flours do not bother gluten-sensitive people.

Although they make nutritious food products, these substitutes fail to give foods the desirable characteristics of gluten-containing flour. Made from corn and rice, foods tend to dry out on standing; made from soybeans, they are heavy, moist, and may have an objectionable beany flavor. The foods the gluten-sensitive person must eat leave much to be desired.

Illness Caused by Gluten

We discussed the scary immediate allergy symptoms caused by wheat. Susceptible people can suffer the anaphylactic hives and breathing blockage of immediate allergy when they eat wheat. We also discussed the delayed symptoms wheat causes, the tiredness and achiness that accompany delayed wheat allergy reactions.

Gluten allergy does not exactly fit either of these two categories. It causes a special illness called celiac disease (also called nontropical sprue or gluten-sensitive enteropathy). We will use the term celiac disease to describe the severe form and gluten intolerance or gluten sensitivity to describe less severe forms.

Different from immediate and delayed food allergies—which do not destroy body tissue—gluten injures the body. In gluten-sensitive people it strips away the inner layer of the intestine like sandpaper.

The "sandpapered" intestine handles food poorly; it struggles to absorb the proteins, carbohydrates, and vitamins from food, and this poor absorption can lead to malnutrition. It poorly absorbs water and other dietary components necessary for health. Much of what a sufferer eats and drinks passes through the intestine and ends up uselessly in the stool.

Gluten Intolerance/Sensitivity in Infancy

Gluten intolerance or sensitivity makes infants dangerously ill. This illness, called celiac disease, appears as soon as gluten is introduced into the diet and can lead to death if not diagnosed.

As it blocks the absorption of foods, it starves infants and children with celiac disease. It makes them look like malnourished victims of a famine—wasted, frail, and feeble, with the protuberant abdomen and thin buttocks of starvation. It gives their stools an awful smell because the undigested fat in the stool stinks. Many children are affected, one in four thousand, but among the Irish, one in five hundred.

In an ironic way, the very severity of this starvation points to the diagnosis. Children look so starved and sick that their condition immediately alerts their doctors that something is terribly wrong. One look at this starved child with thin buttocks and protuberant abdomen and the doctor suspects celiac disease. As the malnourished victims of celiac disease present such a striking picture of sickness, seldom is the diagnosis in doubt.

This ease of diagnosis in infants does not extend to older children and adults who suffer a less severe form of gluten allergy, a condition we are calling gluten intolerance or gluten sensitivity. As you or a loved one may suffer from this less severe form of gluten intolerance, let's look at the problem.

Gluten Intolerance/Sensitivity in Older Children and Adults

An unknown number of people—perhaps few, perhaps many—suffer from the less severe form of gluten sensitivity. Unlike celiac disease, which strikes the very young, they may not notice these less severe forms until the teens or even later in life.

Symptoms may not be those of starvation; they may be tiredness, cramps, diarrhea, or other flulike afflictions that act like delayed food allergy. As many illnesses cause these same symptoms, including other types of allergy, neither doctors nor patients may suspect gluten sensitivity.

This is a tough diagnosis to make; doctors find it difficult to even think of it when they evaluate patients. They more readily think of infectious mononucleosis, fibromyalgia, stress, chronic fatigue syndrome, or other causes of prolonged tiredness and sickness.

I share this difficulty in diagnosing it, and even in thinking of it. As an allergist, I find it easier to look for allergy to dust, mold, or animal dander, which commonly cause these symptoms. My thoughts more easily focus on MALS food allergy, which I see so frequently in my patients, or classic food allergy caused by wheat or other foods and not depending on their gluten content. These other environmental and dietary allergens provoke similar symptoms.

Diagnosis of Gluten Intolerance

Skin tests sometimes help us understand food allergy, and it seems logical that they would help diagnose gluten sensitivity. Unfortunately, they do not help—gluten sensitivity hides successfully from our food skin tests.

The proteins of the gluten that cause this sensitivity, called gliadin proteins, will not dissolve in water, and water is the fluid used to dissolve allergens in our usual skin tests. If we use scratch or injections skin tests to measure food allergy, we cannot measure gluten allergy. A negative skin test to wheat does not mean that one tolerates gluten.

Intestinal biopsy tests. The only way sure way to make the diagnosis of gluten sensitivity is by looking at a piece of the intestinal lining under a microscope. If the lining shows "sandpapering," the patient suffers from gluten intolerance or celiac disease. As this piece of intestine can be obtained only by intestinal biopsy, which is expensive and uncomfortable, we seldom use it in the many patients who suffer the "usual" food allergy symptoms.

Blood tests. One further test may help, checking the blood for antibodies against the gluten. There are a number of antibodies that a medical care professional can search for, each helpful in diagnosing gluten sensitivity.

For all these reasons, those older children and adults who suffer less severe forms of celiac disease may never learn that they must avoid wheat.

Difficulty in diagnosis. The problems of diagnosis we discussed bring us back to the worry I mentioned. How does an allergist identify gluten-sensitive patients from among the many patients suffering chronic flulike symptoms? All the allergist can do is try to keep this diagnosis in mind, especially in the following patients:

◊ patients who continue to suffer in spite of the allergist's treatment
◊ relatives of patients with celiac disease (they may share this illness)
◊ patients with chronic and often poorly defined illnesses such as fibromyalgia, chronic fatigue syndrome, or stress symptoms

Could some of their symptoms be caused by gluten intolerance?

Why Do Some People React to Gluten?

Our knowledge about gluten sensitivity is somewhat limited. We do know that there seems to be a genetic weakness that allows only certain people to react, although the exact identity of this genetic weakness is not clear. However, we do not know what makes gluten so harmful to these people, what leads to the illness called celiac disease. Many experts have tried to explain gluten's power to harm; one or more of these experts may be right.

I'd like to propose an explanation that is peculiar to food allergy. It makes good sense to me.

The gliadin proteins in gluten—the proteins that cause gluten intolerance/sensitivity/celiac disease—are made predominately of one amino acid. Can you guess the identity of this amino acid? The answer is right in the name gluten—it's glutamic acid, the same glutamic acid of monosodium glutamate (MSG). Because we already examined MSG's effect on my MSG-sensitive patients, you should know right away what that means.

This high content of glutamic acid suggests a reason for the illnesses caused by gluten: Could the glutamic acid released from gluten harm the intestine during absorption? I believe that is possible. Could the absorption of this glutamic acid-enriched protein cause tiredness, irritability, headaches, and other symptoms? I wonder.

Does this mean that all people who react to MSG also have gluten sensitivity? Not at all. Many of our MSG-sensitive patients eat wheat without trouble; their genes probably do not predispose them toward gluten sensitivity. Similarly, gluten sensitivity does not necessarily lead to sensitivity to MSG. However, I will try to remember that patients with one sensitivity may also suffer the other.

A Caution

I told you about celiac disease because, as you attempt to understand food allergy, you must include this illness among your thoughts. However, I do not want you to try to diagnose it without help. It is a serious illness.

If you suspect that you suffer from it, consult your primary caregiver. Be tested for other illnesses with similar symptoms. If it appears likely that you react to gluten, take the necessary tests to confirm or deny gluten sensitivity. See the appropriate specialists whom your medical care professional suggests. Do not try to make this diagnosis by yourself.

The preceding discussion of wheat allergy and wheat gluten intolerance prepares us to make the next step: putting together our knowledge about wheat to devise a treatment plan. We will examine treatment next.

Discovering and Managing Your Wheat Allergy

How do you discover if you are allergic to wheat, and if you are, what do you do about it? Let's use our knowledge about wheat to answer these questions.

Are You Allergic to Wheat?

If you react immediately to wheat. If you react quickly after eating wheat, you should have no doubt that wheat causes your symptoms. You may eat a slice of bread or a wheat cracker and start to wheeze or break out in hives. Perhaps you suffer severe stomach pain, your lip swells, or you start to sneeze. Any of these or similar symptoms should immediately focus your attention on the wheat you ate and leave you in no doubt that you suffer immediate allergy to wheat.

If you react to wheat hours after you eat it. As we discussed, delayed allergy to foods can be difficult to diagnose. Many other illnesses make you suffer these same symptoms and, in searching for these other illnesses, you can easily overlook a delayed reaction to wheat. You must think of it to discover it. Therefore, your first step in healing yourself is to think of the possibility.

A Wheat-Free Diet

Your second step is to eat a wheat-free diet for a week and see if your tiredness, achiness, stomach pain, or stuffed nose improves. Then return wheat to your diet for a week. Eat it at every meal. Retry this dietary trial time and again until you are sure of the results. Do you feel better when you avoid wheat and worse if you eat it? If so, you probably are allergic to wheat. However, if you are allergic to wheat, avoiding it may not give you complete symptom relief. You will not gain this relief if, in addition to your wheat allergy, you suffer from a non-allergic illness such as arthritis, Crohn's disease, fibromyalgia, or chronic fatigue syndrome. These diseases often cause symptoms similar to those of delayed food allergy, and their symptoms will persist even though you avoid wheat.

If you suffer from these diseases or from others such as lupus, arthritis, or other nonallergic illnesses, be aware that you also may suffer from allergy, including food allergy. If you do not avoid the foods that make you suffer, your food allergies will combine with these other illnesses to increase your misery.

If you gain even partial relief from avoiding wheat, you should continue to avoid it. You will only gain freedom from pain and discomfort by conquering your illnesses one after another.

If you suffer from other food allergies or from the dust and mold in your home, the same principle applies. Avoiding wheat may give you only partial relief, but this partial relief is welcome. You still need to avoid wheat to achieve your maximal recovery from illness.

Do You Suffer from Gluten Intolerance?

If you suffer from gluten intolerance, you will need to eliminate more than wheat. You also must eliminate from your diet oat, barley, and rye products. As I mentioned, there is some evidence that sensitive people may tolerate some oat. This gluten intolerance diet is a far more restrictive diet than that needed to control wheat allergy, which usually allows you to use oat, rye, and barley as substitutes.

If you suspect gluten sensitivity, explore the possibility by eliminating gluten from your diet. Find a book on gluten elimination at a library or bookstore. Because of the severe dietary restrictions imposed by this diagnosis and the possibility of serious body harm from gluten, involve your medical care professional if you suspect this diagnosis. Never try to diagnose it by yourself.

Managing Your Wheat Allergy

How you manage your wheat allergy depends on how strongly you react to wheat. Your symptoms may be severe, they may be moderate, or they may be mild.

If you react severely to wheat. Perhaps you experience one of the anaphylactic reactions we discussed. If you do, you must not eat wheat; a wheat-free diet is the only treatment possible. Your allergy may not extend into the other grains: oats, rye, and barley. Try them to see if you can use them.

If you suffer moderate to mild wheat allergy. If your wheat allergy is less severe, you do not need to eliminate wheat entirely from your diet. However, you must eat it in moderation so that you consume only the amount you tolerate. Perhaps you can eat a few slices of bread each day or eat wheat cereal in the morning without discomfort. You may find that taking wheat out of your diet for one day allows you to eat it for the next two to four days.

Many of my wheat-sensitive patients tell me that they cannot tolerate whole-wheat foods. However, they tolerate foods made with more processed wheat, such as bread made with white wheat flour. You may share their sensitivity to whole wheat but be able to tolerate white wheat flour, and, if so, will be able to eat some wheat products without trouble.

However, one of my patients notices just the opposite. Perhaps others also tolerate whole wheat but not further refined wheat flour.

Identifying Wheat in Manufactured Foods

Managing your wheat allergy means reading labels to identify foods containing wheat. There are many names for wheat and I have tried to include those you will most likely encounter.

The following labels indicate the presence of wheat protein:

All-purpose flour	High-gluten flour
Bleached flour	High-protein flour
Bran	Semolina
Bread crumbs	Spelt
Bugler	Unbleached flour
Cereal extract couscous	Vital gluten
Durum flour	Wheat bran
Durum wheat	Wheat germ
Enriched flour	Wheat gluten
Farina	Wheat malt
Gluten	Wheat starch
Graham flour	Whole-wheat flour

The following may contain wheat protein:

Cornstarch	Protein
Hydrolyzed vegetable protein	Starch
Gelatinized starch	Vegetable gum
Modified food starch	Vegetable starch
Modified starch	

You will find wheat in instant breakfasts, many baked goods, most baking mixes, pancakes, waffles, and many cereals. Many crackers contain wheat, as do breaded foods, wheat tortillas, pasta, noodles, prepared meat products, hot dogs, and luncheon meats. Look for it in gravies and sauces thickened with flour, and also in cakes, cookies, pies, and other sweet treats. Wheat also can be a component of soy sauce, pretzels, and beer, including nonalcoholic beer.

Controlling Your Other Allergies

You can increase your tolerance to wheat by reducing your other allergies. Watch for symptoms of allergy to other foods and, if you find them, change your diet. Lower your intake of these other foods to the amount you tolerate without symptoms. As your allergy reactions subside with your new diet, you may find that you can eat more wheat.

Lowering your environmental allergy load by lowering moisture, dust, mold, and animal dander levels in the home may similarly allow you more freedom to eat wheat.

Corn

Like wheat, corn occupies a prominent place in our modern diet, and we eat it frequently. Also like wheat, it is a common source of trouble, causing both immediate and delayed symptoms. Some people suffer quickly after they eat it, while others suffer hours later. Those who suffer quick-onset symptoms should have no trouble realizing that corn makes them suffer, but those who suffer later can be very confused.

Corn Protein Food Allergy

We will look first at immediate and delayed symptoms from corn protein—classic food allergy—and then examine how corn also may participate in MALS food allergy.

Immediate Symptoms
If you have immediate allergy to the protein of corn, you can suffer while you eat it or soon after. Within minutes you may develop a reaction similar to hay fever. Your nose swells shut, your eyes itch, and you sneeze. Sinus and migraine headaches may make your face ache or your head throb.

If you suffer from asthma, corn may make you wheeze and short of breath. It can provoke hives anywhere over your body.

These symptoms bother you but do not endanger you; they typically fade away quietly. However, if you react to corn with the anaphylaxis we reviewed earlier, your symptoms frighten you. Quickly you feel your breathing blocked, your head light and dizzy. This quick reaction lets you know that eating corn may threaten your life.

Fortunately, to my knowledge, corn seldom causes these dangerous symptoms. Unlike peanuts, crustaceans, and some other foods, corn's ability to make you quickly and dangerously ill is mercifully limited. Yet, while it seldom causes dangerous immediate symptoms, it frequently causes distressing delayed symptoms.

Delayed Symptoms

I see many patients who react slowly to corn. They suffer typical delayed symptoms—they feel tired and irritable, and they concentrate poorly. Their head hurts, and their joints and muscles ache; their stomach growls and cramps. In other words, they suffer flulike symptoms without end.

With its delayed onset, persistent symptoms, and tendency to strike only when enough corn is eaten to provoke symptoms, patients and doctors often fail to realize that corn is to blame.

Complicating the Diagnosis of Delayed Corn Allergy

Even though I specialize in treating food allergy and should find this diagnosis easy to make, I instead find diagnosing this delayed allergy difficult. It shares its flulike symptoms with many other food allergies that more frequently cause these same symptoms.

Further complicating the diagnosis, foods are not the only cause. Dust mites, mold, pollen, and animal dander allergy commonly cause delayed flulike symptoms. Both the patient and the allergist may direct attention to these other allergies and not think of corn allergy.

We often start suspecting corn only after we find our treatment is not giving the results we expect. Although we have eliminated other foods that cause symptoms and we find and treat dust, mold, pollen, and animal dander allergy, our patients still suffer. Their tiredness, achiness, and other symptoms either remain unchanged or do not subside to the extent that we anticipated.

Realizing that we gave the patient only partial relief, we start thinking of the possibility of wheat or corn allergy. In other words, partial or complete treatment failure makes both wheat and corn allergy prime suspects.

MALS Food Allergy to Corn

Prominent among the MALS food chemicals that cause delayed symptoms is monosodium glutamate (MSG). People sensitive to MSG look for this chemical—in all its various names—on the labels of the foods they buy. They are right to do so. However, they are not right if they think that their only exposure to high levels of MSG is through processed foods such as snacks, soups, and sausages.

Certain unprocessed foods such as tomatoes, mushrooms, and peas also contain high levels of MSG, and sensitive people should limit their consumption of these foods.

Corn and MSG

Corn also contains high levels of MSG. It is easy to visualize how it got there. Over the past few thousand years, farmers planted and grew corn. As they selected the corn seeds to plant next, farmers must have chosen large seeds from strong plants.

They also must have chosen the tastiest seeds, those with superior flavor. How would a plant develop superior flavor? By elevating its level of free glutamic acid. Free glutamic acid not only improves taste, it also makes MSG.

So a warning to those people who are MSG-sensitive: the corn on your grocer's shelves contains elevated levels of MSG. It does not mean that you can't eat it, but watch for symptoms when you do!

Popcorn and Corn on the Cob

Many patients often tell me that although they tolerate boiled corn well, popcorn and corn on the cob trouble them. How many patients react to these foods I do not know, but my discussions with patients tell me that this food sensitivity is not uncommon.

I share these symptoms. If I eat too much corn on the cob or popcorn, I feel ill, and my stomach hurts. This is not the case with corn boiled until it is soft; the boiling seems to eliminate corn's ability to bother me. The corn must be boiled well; if the kernels are still crunchy when I eat them, my stomach hurts. I even find that I can tolerate corn on the cob if it is boiled until the kernels are soft.

How does boiling corn well make it acceptable? Does it boil away the MSG of corn? Does it destroy or remove an allergenic corn protein? I do not know which possibility is more likely; both may be important.

Watch to see if you react to popcorn or corn on the cob. If you do, you still may be able to eat well-boiled corn.

Corn and Alcoholic Beverages

A further tip: if you are corn-sensitive, you may also react to alcoholic beverages made of corn, such as bourbon, some blended scotch whiskeys made partially with corn, and beer that uses corn as one of the brewing constituents. Again, I must speak of my own experiences. I cannot drink any corn-based alcoholic beverage in comfort. I feel sick halfway through a glass of corn-based beer.

You may share my corn sensitivity. If alcohol in moderation makes you sick or headachy, read the label on the alcoholic beverage to find its ingredients. Do not drink beverages not adequately labeled.

Other Corn-Based Foods

Your corn allergy may be restricted to popcorn, corn on the cob, and alcoholic beverages. If so, you may or may not tolerate other corn-based products, such as corn syrup, chips, breakfast cereals, and cornbread.

Corn and Gluten Intolerance/Sensitivity

Although corn has appreciable MSG, its content of gluten is small compared to wheat. It should be safe to eat for the person sensitive to gluten.

The Wheat-Corn Combination

Because of their frequent coexistence, I have learned that at the same time that I look for delayed allergy to corn, I also look for delayed allergy to wheat. I am finding both, especially in those patients with persistent symptoms that respond poorly to our usual treatment.

When corn allergy is mild, my patients easily treat themselves by not exceeding the amount they tolerate. Substituting rice and other grains usually works well. Not so with patients with severe allergy to corn and wheat—their problem is major. Our modern diet relies heavily on these two foods, and completely eliminating them from the diet is a major undertaking. They must eat a diet that is grossly restricted.

If you know that you react to corn, suspect that wheat may also trouble you. Conversely, if you know you react to wheat, suspect that corn may also bother you.

Try restricting your intake of these foods for a week or two and see if your symptoms relent. Reintroduce them to your diet in large quantities to check your findings—notice if your symptoms return. If they return, eat varying amounts until you find your own tolerance to corn and wheat—the amount you can tolerate without suffering.

Wheat-Corn Tiredness

Some of our patients allergic to wheat find that it brings great tiredness. Others find that corn allergy causes this same tiredness. They suffer greatly, dragging themselves through their tasks, trying to study in school, work at their job, or run a home while wishing they could sink into a comfortable bed and sleep. Sufferers bitterly resent their tiredness, and they are right to do so.

Corn and wheat allergy are not the only allergies that cause tiredness, as fatigue is one of the most common symptoms of many types of allergy. It drives many of our patients to seek our help.

Usually I can give them relief. However, some gain only partial relief, and I wonder why. Could my patients' exposure to dust and mold be responsible, especially the often-significant exposures they encounter at home or at work, exposures we cannot change? On the other hand, is delayed allergy to these common foods—corn and wheat—making my patient tired?

Often we find the answer, but sometimes, especially in more complicated cases of allergy, we do not, no matter how hard we try. When we fail, all I can tell my patients is the same advice I give you now:

If you suffer from unreasonable tiredness, beware of delayed allergy to wheat and corn. Experiment with your diet. See if adding or subtracting these foods affects your level of tiredness. If you find that they bother you, reduce your consumption to the amount you can eat without feeling tired. Look closely for other allergic exposures that also bring tiredness.

CHAPTER 6

Preparing to Treat Your Food Allergy

My Patients' Stories

Now you need to put into action the knowledge you learned so you can identify the foods that cause you pain and discomfort and eliminate them from your diet or reduce your consumption of them to the amount you tolerate. We looked at three principles that should guide you in your efforts:

◇ Suspect allergy; you cannot treat your allergy if you do not suspect it.
◇ Do not think that your age protects you from allergy; it doesn't.
◇ You can be allergic to any food, even foods you have tolerated for years.

There are other principles you should know. To help you learn these principles, meet my patients who share your symptoms. Many of these patients suffer from allergic illnesses caused by foods; as we hear their stories, we will discuss other general principles I use in my practice and that you can use to treat your own or a loved one's food allergies.

Some patients suffer complicated food allergies; some do not. The three patients we are about to hear from suffer from complicated food allergies that forced them to change their diets and their lives. Now that you know about MALS and classic food allergies, you will better understand their stories. Their woes will show you how MALS and classic food allergies interact and also will show how these allergies activate physical symptoms as well as symptoms that many consider psychological.

Sue's Story

First we will meet Sue's children, Matt and Ashley. When allergy moved into Sue's house, it toted a suitcase packed with allergy directed against many of the foods we eat daily, foods that make Matt and Ashley sick. In addition to reacting to food, they also react to the ubiquitous dust mites, molds, and pollens that float in the air of their house and in the summer breezes in which they play.

The children have returned to the office so I can learn how they responded to treatment. We started treating Ashley with injections of dust, mold, and pollen six weeks ago, after her skin test showed allergies to almost everything we tested. The test reactions were large, indicating significant allergy.

"She's doing pretty well, Dr. Walsh," Sue replied.

"Tell me about Ashley's diet, Sue." In our previous discussion she told me how hard she worked to feed Ashley a nutritious diet while avoiding all the foods that made her sick.

"It's much like we discussed before," Sue replies. "Ashley still tolerates only a little corn, soy, or rice. Too much and her nose stuffs up and her eyes itch. I can let her have very little sugar or citrus; they do the same. In addition to her itchy eyes and stuffy nose, if I don't watch her diet closely she becomes very irritable and can't concentrate."

Switching my attention to Sue's son Matt I asked, "Are we making progress on Matt's skin, Sue?" Prior to treatment, eczema made Matt's skin as rough and dry as sandpaper, and red with the rash of eczema. I remember his continued itching and the sores his little fingernails dug into his skin. Now Matt's skin feels much softer than before, and there are few scratch marks on it.

"He's much better," Sue said with a smile. "His skin was even better than what you see today. I couldn't get to the office for his last allergy shot, and the rash is coming back. It should get better again soon, now that he receives his shot."

"Do you still have to watch his diet?" I ask.

"Yes, I have to watch it closely. If I don't, his face breaks out in hives, his skin dries out, and he itches until he bleeds. Like Ashley, he can eat soy and corn only if I keep the amounts small and rotate them in his diet. I can give him wheat or sweets if I keep the amount he eats small, but even a small amount of acid foods such as oranges makes him completely miserable."

"Does his mood change with his diet, Sue?" I ask.

"Yes, it does. His mood changes even more quickly and severely than Ashley's. When he gets into foods he shouldn't eat, his irritability and misbehavior become so bad I can't control him. [How often other mothers have noticed the link between behavior and diet.] Yesterday he got into some food—I'm not sure what he ate, but he ran around the house for hours and wouldn't stop even when I threatened him with a spanking."

Barbara's Story

I have treated Barbara for years. Prior to treatment, Barbara's allergies in the spring and fall pollen seasons made her nose run and her eyes itch. Painful headaches visited her daily; many food allergies constricted her food choices. Now, with treatment, she suffers less.

I asked Barbara about these food allergies. She replied, "I still have to watch my diet closely, Dr. Walsh. I still can't eat very much beef, cheese, or potatoes. If I eat pizza, tomatoes, citrus fruits, juices, or foods made with tomato sauce, my whole body swells. My nose blocks off completely, and I get sores in it. Bad headaches start in my nose and travel in a band around my head to my ears, and the pain is awful."

"I'm also very sensitive to wine. Once I drank a sip of champagne and all of a sudden my shoes felt tight. I looked down and saw that my legs and feet had swollen grotesquely, like huge sausages."

Barbara ended her description by describing what happens when she eats salty food. From head to foot, she bloats.

"Once I was in the hospital and the doctors and nurses refused to believe I was so sensitive to salt. They gave me an IV with a normal saline [saltwater] solution. The next morning my mother came to the hospital and was shocked to see me all bloated up. She told the nurses that I looked terrible, all swollen and puffy.

"They didn't believe her until they weighed me and found I gained eleven pounds overnight." With a wry smile she said, "They sure got to work fast then, changing the salty IV to one without salt."

Barbara's story troubles me greatly, and I imagine it also troubles you.

What Our Patients' Stories Tell Us

I'd like to explain what our three patients were telling us and how their experiences guide us to further principles of allergy diagnosis and treatment.

Matt, Ashley, and Barbara suffer immediate and delayed food symptoms. These symptoms are common; my patients suffer them frequently. Every day I treat many who react quickly or slowly after eating. My experience with these patients convinces me that food allergy occurs often.

Comparing symptoms. Symptoms caused by both of these food allergies are similar, and for good reason. Neither actually makes the symptoms our patients suffer. Our immune system makes these symptoms; food allergies merely pull the trigger that sets off the immune system. The bullet that emerges from the immune system gun contains its chemicals, antibodies, and immune cells. This bullet causes the suffering we call food allergy symptoms.

In many ways, MALS food allergy is more important than classic food allergy, and we have a hint of this in our patients' stories. It is the eight-hundred-pound gorilla who came to dinner and sits wherever he desires. As a group, my patients suffer more frequently and severely from the chemicals of foods than from their proteins.

When thinking about allergy symptoms, remember that they can be delayed, arising hours after eating. In MALS food allergy the chemicals in many foods cause these delayed symptoms, and they strike only when you ingest an overload of these chemicals; a tiny bit won't bring trouble. The same is true in delayed classic food allergy.

On the other hand, symptoms can appear quickly. MALS symptoms can strike as quickly as those of immediate classic food allergy. For very sensitive patients, an excessive amount of chemical-laden food can bring quickly appearing distress. In classic food allergy, overload is not necessary; in some conditions, such as anaphylaxis, a tiny taste of shrimp or peanut can be threatening.

Chemicals or proteins cause the symptoms. MALS symptoms differ from classic symptoms, not in how they appear but in what causes them.

Proteins of food cause classic food allergy. In foods such as milk, wheat, carrots, or shrimp, proteins specific to each food trigger the allergic symptom. In contrast, proteins do not cause food chemical symptoms. My patients find that simple chemicals such as refined sugar trigger their reactions. They also can react to food acids, as well as the amino acids found in MSG and low-calorie sweeteners. When they eat or drink more of these chemicals than they tolerate, they suffer.

The Meaning of Sue's Story

Now let's examine what our patients are telling us. Sue's story about her children shows that allergy affects them seriously. As you read about Matt and Ashley's symptoms, you noticed that they suffer both physical and psychological discomfort.

Ashley's physical discomfort includes nose stuffiness and eye itch, symptoms readily acknowledged as caused by allergy by medical caregivers and patients. However, these same people often fail to realize that allergy can cause her irritability and lack of concentration. Many find it much more comfortable and popular among their peers to attribute these symptoms to stress, defective family relationships, or when she is older, to school phobia. Food allergy does not always cause these conditions but should be considered when they exist.

Matt's main physical symptom is his eczema, which is severe when he eats an uncontrolled diet. Eczema is well known to be associated with allergy. However, his mood swings to irritability, misbehavior, and even hyperactivity are frequently attributed to disorders of the psyche instead of disorders of the diet.

We will talk more of disorders of mood and emotions in the section "Can Allergy Affect Your Mood and Emotions?" later in this chapter.

A look at the foods involved. Now that you know about MALS and classic food allergies, you can see that both are involved. Like two programs on your PC running at the same time, these two allergy programs run at the same time on Ashley and Matt's internal computers.

Ashley's classic food allergy involves her reaction to soy and rice. Neither contains excess chemicals of MALS food allergy. Her reaction to corn may be either classic or MALS—directed against corn's MSG content or its protein. Sugar and citrus belong solely to MALS food allergy.

Matt's food allergies are similar, although he is not so sensitive to corn.

The Meaning of Barbara's Story

Barbara bears a great burden. Her diet is painfully constricted because of her uncomfortable nasal congestion and sores, tormenting headaches, and unusual body swelling. In fact, her swelling is more than unusual, it is extraordinary; I do not recall another patient who swells and bloats as Barbara does. Her tale of swelling in the hospital from the IV containing salt water is unmatched, and I can see how her caregivers ignored her plea that they spare her the salt.

As with Matt and Ashley, Barbara's food allergies involve both MALS and classic allergies. Classic food allergy makes her react to beef, and MALS makes her react to the acids in citrus fruits and juices, the MSG in cheese, and the MSG/acids in tomatoes, wine, and pizza. The salt reaction fits neither food allergy and probably results from salt aggravating her tendency to bloat.

You can see the interplay of MALS and classic food allergies in Matt, Ashley, and Barbara's stories. We also saw how Matt and Ashley suffered both physical and psychological symptoms from foods. Your food allergies may be the same, and I hope that these stories can help you understand your own suffering.

Putting It All Together

If you find yourself a little overwhelmed by all our talk of immediate and delayed symptoms and by classic and MALS food allergies, you might benefit from reviewing these factors while hearing the story of another patient.

Let's start this review by listening to Joe's story—it should help to build your confidence that you can treat your own food allergy. You can do it like Joe did it. He discovered his food allergies by himself, before he first came to our office. His wisdom and his efforts impressed me and should impress and reassure you that you can follow his path to health.

Before we meet Joe, let me tell you a little about him.

Bad things shouldn't happen to people like Joe. He's paid his dues to society—worked at his job, paid his taxes, and raised a family. In retirement, he expected pleasant years and good health as repayment for his virtuous life. However, his retirement years were not pleasant and his health was not good; stomach pain tormented him.

The pain started seven years before his visit to my office, and it seemed tied to his diet. By altering his diet and watching for the foods that made his stomach hurt, he identified food after food that caused pain. Unfortunately, as he found each of these foods, his diet contracted, finally shriveling to bread, bananas, rice, fish, and canned vegetables. Anything else caused terrible stomach pain accompanied by a symptom salad of pronounced nausea, dizziness, and retching.

In addition, some foods acted like potent laxatives: chocolate, alcoholic beverages, too many fruits, and rich ice cream. They made him run to the toilet.

Joe visited many doctors; he endured many tests and examinations. Prior to visiting us, his last evaluation was at a world-famous clinic. There, his blood tests were normal, as was an examination of his intestines with an endoscopy tube. Surprisingly, nobody paid much attention to his history of food allergy; they did not urge him to see an allergist.

Although doctors dismissed his suspicions, Joe believed that foods caused these prostrating illnesses. His belief seems likely to be true when matched with his family history. Two of his children react badly to sugar, coffee, wheat, and dairy products—a warning flag that food allergy stalked his family.

He decided to take matters into his own hands and investigate his suspicions. Let's follow the steps he took toward diagnosing and avoiding his food allergy; we can adopt many of them to solve our own problems.

Using Guidelines to Treat Ourselves

Through our previous discussions of guidelines and principles of diagnosis and treatment, you are gaining skill in managing food allergy. We will review these guidelines and principles before examining Joe's story and then see how Joe unknowingly applied them to his self-treatment.

When we first looked at diagnosis and treatment, we discussed the following guidelines:

◊ No illness is allergy until it is diagnosed as such by your primary-care provider.
◊ A nonallergic illness does not preclude allergy.
◊ Never ignore environmental allergy in diagnosing food allergy.
◊ Never ignore food allergy in diagnosing environmental allergy. Explore both food and environmental allergy in every patient.
◊ Attack overpowering food allergy by attacking environmental allergy.
◊ Acidic foods, MSG, aspartic acid, and refined sugar generate the most important food allergies.
◊ Temper your diet with common sense.
◊ Don't be discouraged.

Then we discussed these principles of diagnosis, principles that can remove roadblocks to diagnosing your allergies:

◊ Suspect allergy; you cannot treat your allergy if you do not suspect it.
◊ Do not think that your age protects you from this allergy; it doesn't.
◊ You can be allergic to any foods, even foods you have tolerated for years.

When we covered immediate and delayed allergy to foods, we discussed the following principles of treatment:

◊ Eliminate foods that bother you severely.
◊ Rotate your foods.
◊ Bring new foods into your diet.
◊ Correct your environment.
◊ Continue to learn.

I want to reexamine and expand on all of these guidelines and principles while we look at Joe's story. Your increasing knowledge of food allergy will help you to understand this expansion and use it in your own care.

Expanded General Principles of Treatment

◊ Suspect allergy.
◊ Realize that there are two types of food allergy.
◊ Look for both immediate and delayed symptoms.
◊ Eliminate foods that bother you severely.
◊ When the foods that bother you cannot be removed:
    Rotate the foods you eat.
    Bring new foods into your diet.
    Do not eat more than you tolerate.
◊ Correct your environment.
◊ Continue to learn.

Suspect Allergy

We covered this subject before and we will cover it again because of all our principles, it is the most basic. To treat allergy, whether caused by the diet or the environment, you must first suspect it. If your medical care professional does not suspect it, then you must suspect it, or you will be condemned to live with its pain and discomfort if you suffer from the allergy.

Many of my patients suffered years of pain and discomfort because nobody suspected allergy. Many of these patients, although they suspected food allergy, allowed someone else—at times their doctors—to persuade them that they were wrong. Someone told them that allergy was a figment of their imagination and made them stop thinking. Don't you be like that. If you suspect allergy, hold on to that suspicion like a bulldog clamped to a trouser leg.

Joe suspected allergy. Several clues pointed to this possibility. I mentioned clue number one: his family history was positive—two of his children were forced to exclude foods from their diets that made them sick. The second clue: he underwent competent medical evaluation that found no other cause of his illness. Both of these clues certainly suggest allergy.

Joe's experiences bring up a cautionary note that is part of our guidelines:

◊ No illness is an allergy until it is diagnosed as such by your primary medical caregiver.

Like Joe, see your primary medical caregiver for evaluation before suspecting or acting on your suspicions about allergy. An illness not connected to allergy may be causing your symptoms. If you fail to detect or treat this other illness, you may suffer.

When tests do not show the cause. This second clue—no other cause found—is especially important because it immediately suggests allergy. Allergy hides itself from stethoscopes, blood tests, or X rays. As in Joe's case, test results often miss it.

When you are sick and X rays and blood tests do not give a reason for this illness, you should ask yourself, "What common illness does not show up on tests?" One answer: allergy. It is common—up to 50 percent of us suffer from mild or severe forms, often without suspecting them. If you combine allergy's common occurrence and its ability to hide from tests, you gain the following guide to suspecting allergy:

If tests are normal but symptoms persist, suspect allergy.

When tests show another illness. But even if tests reveal a nonallergic illness, don't drop your suspicions about allergy. Another patient, Betty, is a good example of combined illnesses. Betty suffers from hypothyroidism and multiple sclerosis. We would never have had the chance to treat her allergic nasal congestion and sinus and migraine headaches if her doctor had allowed her nonallergic illnesses to blind him to her allergies. If he had, she would still be stuffy, wheezy, and miserable with head pain.

Be like Betty's doctor—suspect that allergy is complicating other illnesses. Like a bully, it delights in attacking areas of the body weakened by other illnesses. It attacks the joints of patients with arthritis, the intestines of sufferers of Crohn's disease or ulcerative colitis. Recognizing and treating allergy quiets these nonallergic illnesses.

These thoughts suggest another guide to suspecting allergy:

Do not let a nonallergic illness blind you to the presence of allergic illness. They often coexist.

Following these two guides allows you to suspect allergy, even when it tries to hide from you.

Once you suspect allergy, you are ready to find and treat it. To help you do this, the next guide springs readily to mind:

When you suspect allergy, remember that the diet can be a major source of symptoms.

Realize That There Are Two Types of Food Allergy, and Look for Both Immediate and Delayed Symptoms

I combined these two principles because they act together. Knowledge of types and symptoms is so important that I wanted to mention both together.

Knowing that food symptoms can be caused by the MALS or classic food allergy helps you find the offending foods. Watching for both immediate and delayed symptoms will prevent you from being fooled if they take a long time to develop.

Remember that delayed symptoms may start long after you leave the table. The headaches or joint pains you wake with in the morning may arise from the wheat, corn, or MSG-containing food you ate last night. How confusing!

Confounding the confusion of these hidden slowpoke reactions, people suffering delayed symptoms typically react to many foods, not just one, and the affected sufferers need to consume an overdose of these foods or beverages before illness strikes.

With your knowledge, the complexity of delayed symptoms should not make you despair! You should also be comfortable with the thought of two types of food allergy. You know that these symptoms and allergies exist. You can find the foods involved. Be brave, be determined, be persistent. Find them!

Eliminate Foods That Bother You Severely

You know which foods to remove if you suffer immediate food symptoms. If you react strongly to shrimp, nuts, or other foods, eliminate them from your diet.

You will find it more difficult to find the foods you need to remove if your symptoms develop slowly. To find these foods, whether they are part of classic or MALS food allergies, you will need to use elimination diets.

Start by eliminating MALS foods. Start your investigation by removing the foods with large amounts of the MALS chemicals—they are commonly involved. Follow the two-week adult and child allergy elimination diet described earlier. It eliminates the foods that contain excess MSG, low-calorie sweeteners, refined sugar, and food acids.

During this two-week elimination diet, review your symptoms to see if you feel better. If so, you have diagnosed your MALS food allergy. If doubts remain, return these foods to your diet to see if your symptoms flare. If still unsure, repeat the elimination and return of foods.

Once you know which foods bother you, you can learn to limit your consumption of them to the amount you tolerate well.

If necessary, follow an elimination diet for delayed food allergy. If avoiding the foods of MALS food allergy does not end your headaches, rashes, or joint or abdominal pains, you need to think of classic food allergy, with its delayed reactions to milk, wheat, other foods, or multiple foods. These delayed food allergies occur frequently in allergic people (although not as commonly as MALS food allergy).

If you suspect that one or more of these foods cause your symptoms, eliminate them from your diet. Do you feel better? If so, return them to your diet and see if your symptoms return. If they do, you have found the foods that cause your illness.

When You Cannot Remove the Foods That Bother You

Rotate the foods you eat.

Bring new foods into your diet

Do not eat more than you tolerate.

Rotation works only for classic food allergy; MALS allergy requires lowering the amount of chemicals in your diet. Bringing new foods into your diet and not eating more than you tolerate help relieve both food allergies.

When Mother Nature made immediate classic food allergy's symptoms, she gave them excellent memories. They remember the foods that activate them and quickly punish you when you eat these foods. However, the memories she gave the slow-onset symptoms of delayed classic food allergy are atrocious.

She gave them lazy, scatterbrain memories that do not start to work until you eat a food for one, two, or three days; then it rouses itself to make your day miserable. It quickly forgets to torment you if you avoid the food for a day or so. This avoidance is called rotating your foods, and it works.

Rotate the foods you eat. For instance, if beef hurts your stomach and you eat beef for several days, you wake up your delayed allergy to beef protein, and it cramps your intestine or hurts your head at your next beef meal. However, if you substitute fish, fowl, or pork for a day or two, it forgets your beef allergy. Back to sleep it goes. Once you return it to sleep, you can again eat beef for another day or two without suffering cramps.

In many people, delayed classic food allergy involves all the foods in the diet—I call it global food allergy—and these people must rotate all their foods and beverages. Alternatively, they can, as in milk allergy, consume them daily in small amounts that avoid triggering symptoms. This also works well.

If you suspect that many proteins of classic food allergy cause your delayed symptoms, rotate your diet. Drop any habit that involves eating the same food every day—no peanut butter sandwich for lunch each day, no apple a day to keep the doctor away.

To assist rotation, bring new foods into your diet to expand the number of foods you eat. The more foods you ingest, the less chance you will eat enough of any one of them to set off those stomach cramps (or headaches, rash, or tiredness). If your symptoms subside, continue to rotate your foods. You will soon learn from experience how often you can include any particular food in your diet so you can feel the best you can feel.

Correct Your Environment

In thinking about correcting your environment, think of children on a playground. They can teach you much about your food allergy as they play a game of "pile on." In this game, one child is wrestled to the ground and all the other children pile on top until they form a mound of little squirming bodies, one on top of another. The playground supervisor hurries to the pile, peels one child after another off the pile, and finally frees the child trapped on the bottom.

Your food allergy acts like these children. When you react to multiple foods, you are the child wrestled to the ground. Then the food allergies all pile on you and trap you at the bottom of the heap. As you groan, squished under this load of food allergies, you realize that unlike the children on the playground, no teacher will help you. You must free yourself. You must peel off your pile one food allergy after another. You do this by identifying these foods and limiting the amount you eat. If you react severely to them, you must cast them out of your diet.

More Than Food

However, you will not truly free yourself unless you realize that some of the allergies piled on you are not food allergies. In many cases food allergy forms only the top layer; the bottom layers—the mischievous instigators—contain your allergies to dust, mold, pollen, or animal dander; they magnify your food allergy. You must also peel them off the pile if you will free yourself from pain and discomfort.

Remember the stories of Matt, Ashley, and Barbara. Each suffered significantly from foods, but they also suffered from the dust mites, mold, pollen, and pets in the environment. Only when they controlled these environmental allergies *and* their food allergies did they feel well.

For you to feel well, you must understand the importance of correcting troubling home, school, and work exposures. Use this thought as a guide in your self-care, a guide to free you from the bottom of the pile:

To relieve the suffering brought on by complicated food allergy, always aggressively attack any allergies to the environment.

Continue to Learn

This principle needs no further explanation. Our patients continue to learn more about their allergies. By reading this book, you also show your ability and desire to learn. Keep learning. And in this regard, let's return to Joe's story.

"It started some time ago, when my doctors couldn't find any reasons why I felt so miserable. I wondered if something in my diet could be giving me all this trouble. I went to the bookstore and started to read books about food allergy, and I came across your diet in *Food Allergies*.

"I followed the diet, eliminating the foods and beverages as you advised [foods that cause MALS food allergy]. My stomach pains disappeared and I stopped feeling so sick and dizzy. As long as I watch my diet, I feel much better."

With a sad look he continued, "I have to avoid many foods that I really like. Chocolate, alcoholic beverages, too many fruits, and rich ice cream make me feel sick quickly after I eat and drink them."

I asked, "From the diet you learned that you must limit your intake of refined sugar, citrus, MSG, and low-calorie sweeteners. Do you need to avoid other foods?"

"Yes," he replied after a pause. "Before I found the foods that really cause my symptoms, I had eliminated many foods from my diet that were not bothering me. Now I can eat many of these foods, and their addition makes my diet much healthier.

"If I rotate the foods I can eat, I feel much better. You and I wondered if I also had delayed food symptoms, but I haven't noticed delayed symptoms. If I react to foods, I always do so within minutes after I eat. By the way, Dr. Walsh, I followed your suggestions and looked for problems in my home that could make my food allergies worse. I made changes, and they really helped. I also notice that my food allergies are worse in the summer pollen seasons, so I really watch my diet during the summer. I'm staying indoors in air conditioning on high-pollen days, and I am going to get pollen allergy shots to make summer easier."

Joe's story proves that a person with no medical training but with "street smarts" and self-acquired knowledge of food allergy can overcome a miserable condition. He resolved a situation that looked hopeless. By his own study and thought, he had followed the steps we discussed.

I have the utmost confidence that you can do the same.

Be Encouraged

Your food allergy is as treatable as any other medical illness. To treat it effectively, you must assume the role of your own primary therapist. To do this, you must understand your food allergy. And make no mistake, only you can understand your food allergy.

No one else reacts to foods the way you react. By observing how you react, you can determine which foods you must completely avoid, which ones you can eat in limited quantities, and which foods bother you so little that you can eat them freely.

Once you learn about your food allergies, you begin to understand yourself. You become your own doctor; you make the informed decisions that allow you to avoid the foods that make you suffer. Your understanding is the first and most important step you can take toward relieving this burden you carry.

Can Allergy Affect Your Mood and Emotions?

"Why did you come to me for treatment?"

This question is so important it rates its own name: "the chief complaint." The main symptom affecting our patient. As practicing doctors, we know that to serve our patients well, we must understand the chief complaint. It points to the symptom most bothersome to our patient and allows us to aim our treatment to relieve this symptom.

Most of our patients answer this question readily, describing decidedly distressing symptoms such as painful sinus or migraine headaches, uncomfortable nasal blockage, terribly itchy skin rash, far too many colds, or lots of abdominal cramps with diarrhea. Other patients hesitate—they seem unable to select any one symptom so troublesome that it forces them to seek our help.

Being moderately slow to see the obvious (some of my "friends" describe my powers of observation less charitably), it took me a long time to realize why they hesitate. Although they may suffer from headaches, stuffiness, rash, colds, or cramps, these are not their worst symptoms. Something else bothers them more—tiredness, irritability, listlessness, and difficulty concentrating. These are disorders of mood and emotions.

How Allergy Affects Mood and Emotions

When I ask my patients why they hesitate to mention their tiredness or irritability, their answers seem hesitant; they look uncomfortable. Again, it took a long time before I understood why. Now I realize that the hesitation and discomfort arise from our social training.

From early life we are conditioned to deny feelings of tiredness, irritability, and listlessness. After all, are these not signs of the inadequate person, the complainer, the person who fails under the strains and stresses of life?

Perhaps these are good signs of troubles of the psyche in some people, but not in people suffering from allergy. Their tiredness, irritability, listlessness, and difficulty concentrating arise not from laziness or defective psychological coping mechanisms. They arise from the nature of their illness. To explain this, it helps to return to our thought that allergy makes us feel like we have the flu.

When the flu virus invades our bodies, it activates the body's infection defense—the immune system. Once activated, the immune system floods the bloodstream with defensive proteins (antibodies) and defensive blood cells (including white blood cells and lymphocytes), plus many immune chemicals that fight germs.

As we saw, the virus does not makes you snivel into a Kleenex. It is only the trigger that shoots the immune-system gun, triggering this barrage of antibodies, defensive cells that rampage through your bloodstream. This immune response drains your energy and makes you nasty.

Allergy acts like this virus. It triggers the immune system's senseless attack, bringing on your tiredness, listlessness, irritability, and gloominess. These disorders of mood and emotions are normal reactions to your allergies, and you share them with millions of Americans. Unfortunately, sometimes they overwhelm you.

Therefore, although you have been conditioned from early life to be a brave soldier and not complain, it's really okay to tell doctors about it. It's not your fault, and you deserve help.

Allergy and Irritability

I estimate that more than half of our patients suffer distressing mood and emotion changes when they suffer significant allergy symptoms. Irritability often wells up, and a few examples among many show how this irritability handicaps our patients.

Example one: I asked, George, a longtime patient and friend—who calls a spade a spade—what symptoms tell him that he needed his next allergy shot. With a grimace (and good humor), George mumbled in his usual gruff voice, "My family tells me to go get my shot because they say I get nasty and unpleasant to live with."

Example two: another story comes from a mother and shows that irritability is not restricted to adults. Recently she brought her son Josh for treatment of his sneezing and nasal congestion episodes. Actually, his stuffiness was rather mild and his sneezing unremarkable. However, another symptom was bad: whenever these episodes started, he became aggressive and impossible to discipline; for several days family life became "pure hell."

Certainly, allergy poisons Josh's mood, roils his emotions, and penalizes his family. He deserved whatever help we can offer.

Allergy and Depression

What about that most severe alteration of mood and emotions—depression? Can allergy cause depression?

No. I do not think allergy causes depression, but—as it does with Crohn's disease and fibromyalgia—it makes the underlying condition worse. Are you surprised that they coexist in the same person? Don't be; both allergy and depression are common, and inevitably many people susceptible to depression also suffer from allergy. To put it another way, many allergic people also suffer from depression. These unfortunate people find their depression harder to battle while their allergy makes their noses stuffy, their heads hurt, and their stomachs ache.

When the flulike tiredness, listlessness, and irritability of allergy accentuate the melancholy of depression, our patients find misery doubled. To give them real relief, we allergists must direct our skills and efforts to treating allergy to the best of our ability.

Food Allergy and Mood

In our examples, I pointed out how pollen, dust, and mold sensitivities affect mood. Can food allergy do the same? Many doctors may say no, but my observations tell me the answer is yes. For instance, listen to Betty's and Lois's stories.

After ten years of treating Betty, I have come to appreciate and admire her warm personality and ever-ready smile. In spite of her cheerfulness, she has suffered much. Prior to starting treatment, she experienced daily painful headaches, a constant stuffy nose, wheezing, and far too many colds.

Allergy injections give her much relief of these painful and uncomfortable symptoms, especially after she moved from a musty old house. But the viral heart infection that laid her low increased her discomfort. In addition, her job forced her to work in two separate buildings where mustiness swelled up her throat, choked off her voice, and labored her breathing. She had to leave both jobs to regain her health.

One sick building was an old school building converted into a factory, where the employees were forced to use buckets to collect rainwater dripping from a leaky roof. It must have been mold hell.

Betty describes her food allergies. "I must avoid many foods, including sugar, MSG, excess citrus, and diet beverages. When I eat or drink them, I feel bloated and nauseated. I then feel very tired and drowsy."

As you saw, many of our patients react to these foods in the same way, so her observations are no surprise. However, the answer to my next question surprised me greatly when I asked it in the past, and it may surprise you today.

"Betty, do any other foods trouble you?"

Again she answered in the affirmative, "Yes. Beef, milk, and whole-wheat bread [which reacted positively on our skin tests] also make me very nauseated, and I'm so tired I can't wait to go to bed. And," she said with some reluctance, as I am sure she thought we would not believe her, "I used to be depressed when I ate beef and drank milk. I didn't realize that they were problem foods for me. A small piece of beef made me feel sluggish, bloated, and depressed."

Betty then tells us that her mother suffers similar depression when she eats these same foods. As with Betty, her mother's depression returns each time she eats them.

Now you know why I was surprised. I found it hard to accept the thought that foods cause depression.

Let me introduce you to another patient whose story agrees with Betty's.

After five years of allergy injection treatment, Lois had stopped taking shots. Unfortunately, daily headaches and repeated respiratory infections returned when we stopped injection treatment. These symptoms worsened when she moved to an apartment where the previous tenant's dog had repeatedly soiled the carpet. She and I agreed that the carpet had to go and that she needed to return to treatment.

Lois is an intelligent and prudent person; let's listen to her response as to whether she has noticed any foods that cause her to be depressed.

"Yes. I suffer intense depression from eating corn, MSG-flavored foods, aged cheese [naturally high in MSG], and acid foods."

"What about oranges?" I ask.

She replies, "With oranges, my spirits just plunge."

Mood, Emotions, and Delayed Food Allergy

There is one way in which delayed food reactions differ from immediate reactions. The former possess a unique power to wickedly touch emotions and mood. Before discovering their food allergies, many of my patients believed that their dark mood and emotions signaled psychological illness. An example of this is our next patient, Leo. His story will amaze you and show you how food allergy profoundly affects mood and emotions.

I have treated Leo for years, and he needs all the help I can give him. He suffers from frequent and painful headaches. Although his need for relief is great, at first our help was minimal. He spent many days in pain.

Leo is a cheerful and polite college student. We talk about his allergies and our treatment.

"My chiropractor diagnosed a wheat allergy. I took the wheat out of my diet, I felt wonderful then, and I still feel wonderful. My headaches are gone.

"The other day I ate some wheat bread and about eight hours later I felt sick. Not only did my head hurt, I also felt tired, irritable, and depressed. You know, before I stopped eating wheat I had many days when I couldn't think well and couldn't get anything done. On those days, I felt so depressed that I worried that I needed medicine for depression. Now, as long as I don't eat wheat, I don't feel that depression."

I confess that I missed Leo's delayed wheat reaction. But my failure illustrates the point I am trying to make: *we underdiagnose delayed reactions to foods!*

If I, a specialist in food allergy, can miss it, other doctors with less interest, training, and experience also can miss it. So when someone tells you that food allergy is rare, allow a little doubt to creep into your mind. Is it really rare or, more likely, common but not diagnosed? I think the true answer is the latter.

Leo's story also illustrates a point I have mentioned before: you can find your own food allergies without consulting an allergist. Another medical caregiver blessed with insight into and familiarity with food allergy, like Leo's chiropractor, may help you, or you may help yourself through your own good observations.

Leo's story also starkly demonstrates the malignant effect that food allergy, especially delayed food allergy, can exert on the mood and emotions. In my experience, it does so commonly.

Conclusions and Questions

The stories of George, Josh, Betty, Lois, and Leo (and many, many others) lead me to certain conclusions but also lead to many questions. Among the conclusions:

◊ Irritability, tiredness, grogginess, and listlessness can result from allergy; patients should not be ashamed to admit these symptoms.

◊ Not all depressed people suffer from allergy. However, some do. When these illnesses coexist, both deserve treatment.

How often do allergy and depression coexist? How can foods worsen depression? How often do they worsen depression? Should we be looking for food allergy in depressed patients? To these questions, I do not have the answers.

Although these questions bring frustration, they also show the fascination of allergy. It affects millions. It encompasses many illnesses and, like an unexplored wilderness, much remains to be discovered. The exploration will be difficult but engrossing, and the discoveries promise to be of unquestioned value.

The Rotation Diet

A rotation diet varies the foods in your diet so that you do not eat them every day. Many of my patients use food rotation or a rotation diet and gain great relief of their symptoms. However, others gain no relief because food rotation, although it helps relieve symptoms of classic food allergy, has certain limitations. It does not help relieve symptoms of MALS food allergy. Limiting the MALS chemicals in the diet helps relieve MALS food allergy. In addition, people suffering classic allergy to one or a few foods do not need to rotate their diets; they simply need to limit their consumption or completely avoid these few foods.

In spite of these limitations, a rotation diet is one of the most useful tools we use to treat classic food allergy where multiple food allergies are involved. It especially helps those who suffer from "global" food allergy. (People with global food allergy react to all the foods they eat. Surprisingly, this is not an unusual pattern of allergy.)

Although multiple food allergy seems to be a horrific mistake of nature—incompatible with life—it really isn't. Many of my patients react to multiple foods and do just fine as long as they rotate the foods they eat. By not eating the same foods daily, the diet is shifted before repetitive eating of the same foods triggers the immune system.

Starting a Rotation Diet

How do you rotate the food in your diet? Any way you want to. There are many books on rotation diets, and you can follow them. Any dietitian will help you. On the other hand, you can decide to use your good common sense and not eat the same foods day after day.

Some general guidelines:

1. Eliminate monosodium glutamate.
2. Do not use low-calorie sweeteners.
3. Limit your intake of refined sugar and acidic foods.
4. Try to include a variety of fresh and nutritious foods in your diet.

In other words, do not let your diet change lure you into a high-MALS diet—you may end up substituting MALS symptoms for classic food allergy symptoms.

Shop at your nearby food cooperatives, whole-foods markets, or the health foods section of your local grocery store. They offer healthy foods we eat too infrequently, alternate foods to add to our conventional wheat/corn/milk diets.

Ideas for a Rotation Diet

The following is meant to suggest foods that you can rotate into and out of your diet. I have included few of the foods with large quantities of MALS chemicals in this diet; I have alerted you to those that remain.

◊ Do not include foods in this diet that you know you react to.

◊ *Protein* includes meats, poultry, fish, and eggs. You can prepare them in various ways, including roasts, chops, liver and other organ meats, ground meats, soups, broths, and stews. Be sure to avoid MSG flavoring in your foods; look for it under any of its many names.

◊ *Grains and flours* include pastas, breads, cereals whether hot or cold, pancakes, waffles, muffins, cookies, crackers, the starch and flakes of grains, and other preparations. Avoid preparations with excess refined sugar. Look for the alternate grains mentioned below in health food stores if your own grocery does not stock them.

◇ *Fruits* are marked below with an asterisk if they contain higher quantities of citrus and other acids. They may be eaten, but try to limit your consumption to the amount you tolerate if you react to acidic foods.

◇ *Vegetables:* potatoes and tomatoes contain appreciable food acids (foods with excess acids also are marked with an asterisk below) and MSG. Grapes and corn contain appreciable naturally occurring MSG; grapes also contain tartaric acid. Avoid MSG-flavored salad dressing— "when in doubt, eat without."

◇ *Spices:* I included the spices to help you think of flavorings for your meals that do not include MSG. I do not mean to imply that the ones I mention for a particular day are the best spices for the foods of the day.

◇ *Beverages:* Water, milk if you tolerate it, coffee, and tea (without flavoring) are beverages acceptable to the MALS-sensitive person. People not sensitive to MALS chemicals can include other beverages, such as carbonated sodas and high-acid juices.

A ROTATION DIET FOR CLASSIC FOOD ALLERGY WITH SENSITIVITY TO MULTIPLE FOODS

Foods for Day One

Protein	Beef (as hamburger, steak, stew, other), pork (as bacon, chops, sausage, other), venison or other wild game
Grains and flours	Barley, oat, rye, wheat (caution: contain gluten)
Fruits	Melons (including watermelon, cantaloupe, honeydew), grapefruit,* lemon*, lime,* oranges*
Nuts	Almonds, pecans, walnuts
Vegetables	Asparagus, artichoke, beets, garlic, lettuce, okra, olives, onion, spinach, sweet potatoes, Swiss chard
Spices	Chives, cinnamon, cloves, mint, mustard, oregano, paprika, rosemary

Foods for Day Two

Protein	Cod, haddock, halibut, herring, mackerel, salmon, sardines, snapper, sole, trout
Grains and flours	Corn, rice, tapioca
Fruits	Apricots,* cherries,* dates,* figs,* nectarines, peaches, plums,* and prunes*
Nuts	Cashews, macadamia nuts, pumpkin seeds
Vegetables	Alfalfa sprouts, bamboo shoots, beans, bean sprouts, peas, red and green peppers, tomatoes,* white potatoes*
Spices	Bay leaves, cayenne, chili, red peppers, sage, thyme

Foods for Day Three

Protein	Chickens, ducks, eggs, guinea hens, turkeys
Grains and flours	Arrowroot, buckwheat, millet, lima beans, peas, soybeans
Fruits	Apples, mangoes, papayas, pears, raspberries,* rhubarb,* strawberries*
Nuts	Pistachios, soy nuts
Vegetables	Carrots, celery, corn, cucumbers, green beans, lima beans, peanuts, parsnip, pumpkin, squash, water chestnut, zucchini
Spices	Caraway, coriander, fennel, garlic, ginger, turmeric

Foods for Day Four

Protein	Any proteins not eaten on days one through three: crabs, clams, lobsters, scallops, shrimp
Grains and flours	Quinoa, sunflower, teff
Fruits	Avocados, bananas, blueberries,* cranberries,* grapes* and raisins,* pineapples
Nuts	Brazil nuts, chestnuts, filberts, pine nuts, sunflower seeds
Vegetables	Broccoli, Brussels sprouts, cabbage, cauliflower, collard greens, horseradish, kale, radish, rutabaga, turnip, watercress, yam
Spices	Black pepper, cumin, dill, nutmeg, vanilla

Why Describe This Diet?

Its purpose is to help you understand your own food allergy. Once you understand, you can find good references that teach you how to follow a diet that avoids wheat, corn, milk, or other foods that may cause your allergy symptoms. Since these diets are readily available in your local bookstore or on the Internet, I have not provided them for you here.

I have provided this rotation diet for two reasons. First, because rotation is so important to so many people I felt I should provide an example. Second, many of my patients suffer from multiple classic (protein) food allergies at the same time as they also suffer from MALS (chemical) food allergies. To decrease their symptoms, they should rotate foods while avoiding excessive MALS chemicals in their diets.

Must You Follow This Diet without Deviation?

Not at all. This is an unusually strict diet; each day's foods are not repeated the next day. Many patients can eat each of these foods two to three days in a row and avoid them the next day without troubling symptoms. They need only imprecise and even "sloppy" rotation to control their allergy symptoms.

Only a tiny minority of patients need a diet this strict; very few must be so precise and dedicated to the diet. But whether patients need a strict or a lax diet, all should be perfectly capable of devising their own rotation diets. Follow this or a diet of your own arrangement only to the extent that you find necessary to feel well.

Use Your Intuition and Knowledge and Just Do It

As I say good-bye and God be with you as you learn to eat healthier, I'd like to leave you with a thought: the value of your intuition in guiding you. The best way to show you this value is by looking at an often recommended process that does not require intuition. This process is the diet diary. Let me tell you why I think it is misleading if you use it to diagnose and treat a complicated case of food allergy.

My patients often ask me if they should use it, if they should record the foods they eat in a food diary. They could then use the diary to try to discover which foods cause their allergy symptoms. My reply: I discourage searching for food allergy with food diaries; they tend to lead my patients astray.

To help you understand why I discourage food diaries, let's look at the experiences of two patients whose stories illustrate why a diet diary may be wrong for you.

Jack is a pleasant young man who works for the city cutting grass in summer. For Jack, this is not a good job. His summer hay fever symptoms blossom like the weeds his mower cuts—the weed pollen erupts from the cutting blades in a sneeze-filled cloud that makes his eyes swell and his nose plug.

Jack's pollen injections and allergy medication give him partial relief, for which he is grateful. But during the pollen seasons he must also avoid certain foods, and this food allergy is the object of our story.

With a worried expression, Jack starts his story: "The part of my food allergy that frightens me the most is my reaction to peanuts. Even a small taste of peanuts makes my throat close off, and I feel like I'm suffocating. I have been rushed to the emergency room several times by the paramedics after eating foods that I didn't realize contained peanuts."

"Jack, you also told me that you cannot eat certain foods when your hay fever symptoms are bad. "

"In the spring and fall, when my sneezing is really bad, I can't eat acid foods such as tomatoes or oranges. If I do, my eyes swell up so much I can't see, and my nose runs like a faucet. The rest of the year I can eat these foods without any discomfort."

Jack's other food allergy, appearing only during the pollen seasons, makes a food diary liable to error. It may have hidden the diagnosis from him. We will discuss this in a minute, but first let's first hear Joanne's story.

Although Joanne does not react violently, she suffers profoundly.

Joanne is one of our many patients with fibromyalgia and at least a suspicion that she may suffer from Crohn's inflammation of the intestine, a diagnosis sometimes hard to make. When I first saw her, she also suffered from frequent and severe headaches that caused daily pressure pain over her sinuses and migraine headaches that each week brought pulsating pain that bored into her right eye.

Her headaches are far fewer now, relieved by drying the basement of her home to eliminate mustiness and by using medication that helps open her sinuses.

Joanne also suffers from allergy to foods. This is her story:

"I didn't realize how much foods bothered me until we started to look for food allergy while investigating my dust and mold allergy. I was soon to find that food indeed caused me much pain."

"What about sugar, MSG, low-calorie sweeteners, and acidic foods?" I ask.

"MSG causes headaches, and I find I can drink only small amounts of diet soda or my head hurts and the pain is intense. My joints also hurt. I can eat a little sugar, but too much and I feel irritable and my stomach hurts and my joints hurt. Tomatoes and orange juice make my skin itch."

"Joanne, on our last visit a year ago we wondered if corn or wheat may also bother you. What did you learn when you eliminated them and returned them to your diet?" I ask.

"I indeed found that corn bothers me, but only fresh corn like corn-on-the-cob or popcorn, and only if I eat too much. Well-cooked corn is okay. I don't seem to have trouble with wheat.

"By the way, I also found that I do not tolerate lactose very well. Milk with lactose gives me loose stools and gas."

Why a Diet Diary Can Lead You Astray

After meeting Jack and Joanne and hearing their stories, let's see how a diet diary can lead them, or you, astray.

It is often unnecessary. In Jack's case, his reaction to peanuts is so severe and quick-acting that there is no question of the cause. No food diary is necessary.

For a diet diary to be effective, only one or a few foods should be involved. A diet diary is useful if you suspect that one or a few hidden foods cause your symptoms. For my patients who suffer distressing symptoms such as headaches, tiredness, or inability to concentrate, this is seldom the case. They commonly suffer from both MALS and classic food allergies and their allergies involve many foods.

Searching for multiple food allergies with a diet diary is an exercise in frustration. Because so many foods may be involved, you often see no sensible pattern emerging from your list of foods.

For a diet diary to be effective, you should react to a food every time you eat it. However, most food allergies do not strike unless you eat enough of the food to precipitate symptoms. Look at Joanne's experience. She, like many of my patients, reacts to many foods with many symptoms. The foods she reacts to include corn, acidic foods, and diet soda. Her symptoms include itchiness, headaches, irritability, abdominal distress, and muscle and joint aches. She suffers quickly after only a small amount of some foods; she must eat more of other foods before symptoms strike.

She suffers from corn, acidic foods, and diet soda only when she exceeds her tolerance for these foods and beverages. If she consumes an amount she tolerates, she does not suffer. If she paid attention to the days when she did not exceed her tolerance, the diet diary may convince her that she is not allergic to these foods.

For a diet diary to be effective, your symptoms should not be influenced by your environment. A food diary may have prevented Jack from discovering his acidic food allergy. If Jack had pursued a food elimination diet in the winter using a diet diary to record his observations, he would have missed the sensitivity to foods that arises only during the pollen seasons. Once convinced of his ability to eat these foods without suffering, he would have looked no farther, and the acidic foods would make his hay fever symptoms miserable.

To discover the acidic food allergy, Jack needed to know that the possibility existed, that food allergy could appear only while he labored under the burden of environmental allergy—pollen in his case. We told him of the possibility. He found that it applied to him.

The same thoughts apply to Joanne. Her musty basement exposed her to high levels of mite and mold in her home, exposures that worsened the symptoms caused by foods. She needed to clean up her environment and receive treatment for mite and mold allergy. Without these measures, her symptoms would be so severe that a diet change would not help her.

If Joanne had followed an elimination diet and recorded her observations in a diet diary while suffering severe environmental allergy symptoms, her symptom improvement would be minimal. She would have been convinced that she did not suffer from foods.

Why Intuition Is Necessary

Joanne's story shows why she needs intuition to manage her diet. She suffers symptoms caused by many foods of both classic and MALS food allergies. To discover these foods, she needs not a food diary but a knowledge of which foods may cause her symptoms. She also needs an almost intuitive feel for which foods trouble her and how much of these foods she can safely eat each day.

When I listen to the stories of my many patients with food allergies such as Joanne's, I marvel at how they can appropriately select the foods they eat each day. They do it well.

Certainly, on some days they cheat by eating a food they crave but shouldn't eat, a perfectly human failure. On those days, they suffer. However, on most days they do not cheat and eat only those foods they can tolerate, and they feel wonderfully well—tribute to their ability to tiptoe safely through the minefield of their food allergies.

What Makes Intuition Work

Intuition works because of the knowledge my patients gain through their observations and through our teachings. When they combine the knowledge gained through this teaching with intuition, they find that even the most complicated food allergies become manageable.

I believe that our intuition arises from our possession of a very perceptive guardian. It exists in us completely unaffected by the odds and ends of moth-eaten and often mistaken information that clutters our conscious mind's attic.

It disregards wisdom such as "Drink lots of orange juice when you are sick" and "Diet pop allows you to lose weight without harm." It does not believe that "MSG seldom causes sickness." It ignores you when you convince yourself that sugar does not make your muscles spasm and your temper flare. Neither you nor the accepted wisdom of society leads it astray.

Our intuition knows what foods cause us pain and discomfort. If we will listen to it, it will guide us in the foods we should select. It will help us be flexible in our diet, watching our foods closely in seasons when our symptoms peak—the pollen seasons for Jack. It will tell us to cautiously restrict our diet when we work in a moldy building or stir up a cloud of moldy dust working in our gardens.

For our intuition to work most effectively, it needs knowledge. You give it knowledge when you read books on food allergy. You give it indispensable knowledge when you eliminate and reenter foods (avoid and challenge) until you are sure which foods bother you and which ones you can eat without restraint.

Intuition and knowledge will help you control your food allergies and help you feel well.

Listen to my patient Joanne's words. I have learned to treasure her insight and common sense through the years I have treated her. Like most of my patients, her allergy symptoms arise from both the diet and the environment. When I asked her to comment about these symptoms, she carefully considered my request and then replied:

"I suffered for years because my allergy got missed or lost in the shuffle. Although my diarrhea occurred soon after I ate foods, my doctor never thought it might be food allergy. He also did not think that my headaches, chest tightness, or joint swelling and stiffness might be delayed reactions to foods.

"I found it hard to believe that I could react to something that I ate two days ago. Everybody has this misconception that food allergy always happens quickly after you eat and that if you do not suffer right after the meal, it's not allergy. This thought is wrong, and it wasn't until I changed my diet that I started to feel better. "

She went on to say that people should realize that the ultimate responsibility for their allergies rests on themselves. Each person has his or her own special symptoms; each reacts to foods and environmental factors uniquely.

In Joanne's case, these symptoms include diarrhea, chest tightness, headaches, and joint swelling. Some foods bother her more than other foods. This pattern of symptoms and causative foods is unique to Joanne; another patient will suffer differently.

A caller from California had a question that many readers ask. She suffered many of the symptoms that signal food allergy: migraine headaches, abdominal pain, diarrhea, and itchy skin. As is too often the case, her allergist told her that these symptoms were not those of food allergy.

She had found my diet and called to discuss her symptoms. She told me that she had been evaluated by her primary medical caregiver, as I have repeatedly advised you to do. No sign of a nonallergic illness had been found.

When I asked her what happened when she used my diet, her answer distressed me. She had not tried it. She had called to get my permission to try it.

I was distressed, because she did not need my permission to try the diet. She suffered from no medical condition, such as diabetes, that would have made the diet difficult to fit into her daily meals. Eliminating the MALS foods for two weeks would not be dangerous for her. She should have used her own independence and common sense to follow the diet to see if her symptoms subsided.

I truly want you to be your own allergist. To do this, once you have eliminated nonallergic causes of your symptoms, and if no medical illness makes changing your foods dangerous, just do it. You do not need my permission or that of any other caregiver to start your investigation by trying the two-week elimination diet in the section "The Adult and Child Allergy Elimination Diet" in chapter 2. There are plenty of nutritious foods you can eat on this diet, foods containing the vitamins, fiber, minerals, and all the other nutrients so essential to your health. Just do it!

APPENDIX:
QUICK-SERVICE RESTAURANTS

Because we often need rapidly served meals, a large restaurant industry arose to serve nutritious meals in an efficient and timely manner in a clean environment. The names of restaurants in this industry—names such as McDonald's and Burger King—spring readily to mind. They satisfy our hunger and satisfy it well. But when we go to these restaurants, what can we eat?

The biggest problem food-allergic people face in these restaurants is avoiding foods flavored with MSG. Because these restaurants use MSG does not mean the restaurant managers unfeelingly disregard your health—they do not. They use MSG only because they believe it is safe and wholesome and they do not believe it will hurt you, their customer.

Avoiding MSG

At my request, McDonald's sent me the complete list of ingredients of all the foods served at their restaurants. Included in the information was a listing of all their products that contain added MSG and also the products to which McDonald's adds hydrolyzed vegetable protein and other terms that tell you the product contains MSG. Other terms, such as "natural flavoring," mean the product may contain MSG.

Which returns us to the question of which foods my patients may order and which they should avoid at fast-food restaurants. To try to answer these questions, I spent several hours with the McDonald's brochure *McDonald's Food: The Facts*, and below I discuss the foods I believe the food-allergic person should avoid and also those they may order.

Eating at McDonald's

The following information has been supplied by McDonald's. This same information is available by contacting:

McDonald's Nutrition Information Center

McDonald's Corporation

Oak Brook, IL 60523

(630) 623-FOOD

The same information is available at the McDonald's site on the Internet.

Foods and Beverages My Patients Should Avoid at McDonald's

Beverages and desserts containing low-calorie sweeteners or large amounts of refined sugar and the citric acids are easy to recognize and therefore easy to avoid.

Sauces and dressings taste good because they contain large amounts of refined sugar and/or citrus and/or MSG. If you have trouble tolerating MSG and high levels of sugar and citrus, avoid both sauces and dressings.

Foods with MSG Added as MSG at McDonald's

Breakfast Burrito

Breakfast sausage patty (and sandwiches containing sausage)

Sausage Biscuit

Sausage Biscuit with Egg

Sausage McMuffin

Sausage McMuffin with Egg

Pizza Sausage

Soups (all of them)

Foods with MSG Added as Hydrolyzed Vegetable Protein at McDonald's

Big Mac

Other food selections at McDonald's may contain MSG. They are supplied to McDonald's by food manufacturing companies, and these foods contain natural flavors, natural flavoring, or seasoning. They may or may not contain MSG. To avoid possible symptoms, if you are sensitive to MSG, avoid the following foods:

Foods Containing Natural Flavorings That May Contain MSG
Filet-O-Fish
Bacon (except Canadian-style bacon)
French fries
Hash browns
Ketchup
Tartar sauce
Honey mustard sauce
Chicken McNuggets (contains beef extract)
Chicken (for salad)
Croutons
Fat-Free Herb Vinaigrette Salad Dressing
Red French Reduced-Calorie Salad Dressing
Ranch Salad Dressing
Sweet 'N Sour Sauce

Finally, MSG is released by fermentation from protein in the manufacture of cheese, wine, and soy sauce. In most cases the presence of cheese is obvious—such as in a cheeseburger, listed next—and is easy to avoid by ordering a hamburger without cheese. Sometimes the presence of cheese is not so obvious, and these cheese-containing foods, plus food containing soy sauce, autolyzed yeast extract, or wine, make up the following list:

Foods with MSG Added as Cheese, Soy Sauce, Autolyzed Yeast Extract, or Wine at McDonald's
Chef Salad (contains shredded cheese)
Caesar Salad Dressing (contains cheeses and natural flavors)
Sweet 'N Sour Sauce (contains soy sauce)
Arch Deluxe
Arch Deluxe with Bacon
Grilled Chicken Deluxe (autolyzed yeast extract)
Cheeseburger
Quarter Pounder with Cheese

**Foods and Beverages the MALS-Sensitive Person
Can Order at McDonald's**

Now I will change focus and indicate the foods and beverages my patients should be able to tolerate. As always, if a patient has an allergic reaction to a particular food recommended on our diet, this food should be avoided. Although refined sugar is used in some of the products mentioned below, I believe that most food-sensitive patients should tolerate the quantity of sugar contained in the food.

For breakfast:

Egg McMuffin (request it without cheese)

Eggs

Milk, coffee, or water

For lunch or dinner:

Hamburger (with pickles, onion, salt, pepper, and mustard)

Quarter Pounder (same as above)

Mustard

Hot mustard sauce

Mayonnaise (contains lemon juice concentrate)

Margarine

Butter

Garden salad (don't eat the tomato)

Milk or water

Eating at Burger King

For my food-sensitive patients, the problems surrounding food selection while visiting Burger King are similar to those presented by food selection at McDonald's. Avoiding MSG and low-calorie sweeteners plus excess refined sugar and the acids of the citrus group demands careful food selection in each restaurant chain.

To let you know why certain foods on the McDonald's menu are excluded from the list of acceptable foods, we examined the list of ingredients at length. The same ingredients are found in many of the selections at Burger King. To prevent this chapter from becoming too long, I will not repeat the reasons for excluding foods with these ingredients. Instead, I will concentrate on the foods my patients should tolerate while eating at Burger King.

Like McDonald's, Burger King cares about the health of its patrons. To help these patrons select appropriate foods, Burger King provides a pamphlet describing the contents of their foods, and I derived the following information from this pamphlet. You can obtain this same information from a Burger King near you or by checking Burger King's web site.

Foods the MALS-Sensitive Person Should Tolerate at Burger King

Burger/sandwich

Whopper sandwich without ketchup; may use mustard

Hamburger without ketchup

BK Big Fish Portion

Breakfast

Ham

Croissant and biscuit contain sodium caseinate

Beverages

Coffee

Milk

Water

Conclusion

The selection of foods my patients can tolerate at quick-service restaurants is limited and omits many delicious choices. This I regret because I, like you, must choose from this limited selection of foods and avoid many I would love to eat.

I chose McDonald's and Burger King to review because I believe they go out of their way to help the allergic person. The entire list of the ingredients of their foods is easily available, both at their restaurants and on the Internet. A restaurant chain that makes this information so available should be complimented and patronized.

If your sensitivity to MSG is slight, you may tolerate some of the foods I failed to mention; I did include some of the foods that contain small amounts of the food chemicals that cause my patients' symptoms when I judged the amounts too small to cause symptoms. Of course, if you do not react to these chemicals, you do not need to avoid these foods.

To guard against changes in ingredients, ask the restaurant you patronize for the list of ingredients in the foods they serve. Not only will you learn to avoid symptoms, but also your concern about eating foods with MSG flavoring will alert the restaurant that this allergy exists and prompt them to consider making a wider choice of foods available to food-sensitive people.

BIBLIOGRAPHY

Amlot, P. L., D. M. Kemeny, C. Zachary, P. Parkes, and M. H. Lessoff. "Oral Allergy Syndrome: Symptoms of IgE-Mediated Sensitivity to Foods." *Clinical Allergy* 17, no. 1 (1987): 33–42.

Anderson, J. A. "Food-Induced Systemic Reactions and Anaphylaxis." In *Allergy, Asthma, and Immunology from Infancy to Adulthood,* edited by W. Bierman, D. S. Pearlman, G. G. Shapiro, and W. W. Busse. Philadelphia: W. B. Saunders, 1996.

Bell, R. T., ed. "A Commonsense Approach to Lactose Intolerence." *Patient Care* 31, no. 7, (1997): 185–190, 195.

Bierman, C. W., D. S. Pearlman, G. G. Shapiro, and W. W. Busse, eds. *Allergy, Asthma, and Immunology from Infancy to Adulthood.* Philadelphia: W. B. Saunders, 1996.

Blanco, C., T. Carrillo, R. Castillo, J. Quiralte, and M. Cuevas. "Latex Allergy: Clinical Features and Cross-Reactivity with Fruits." *Annals of Allergy* 73, no. 4 (1994): 277–281.

Brehler, R., U. Theissen, C. Mohr, and T. Luger. "Latex-Fruit Syndrome: Frequency of Cross-Reacting IgE Antibodies." *Allergy* 52, no. 4 (1997): 404–410.

Breneman, J. C. "Immunology of Delayed Food Allergy." *Otolaryngology and Head and Neck Surgery* 113, no. 6 (1995): 702–704.

Charlesworth, E. N., A. Kagey-Sobotka, P. S. Norman, L. M. Lichtenstein, and H. A. Sampson. "Cutaneous Late-Phase Response in Food-Allergic Children and Adolescents with Atopic Dermatitis." *Clinical Experimental Allergy* 23, no. 5 (1993): 391–397.

Crowe, S. E., and M. H. Perdue. "Gastrointestinal Food Hypersensitivity: Basic Mechanisms of Pathophysiology." *Gastroenterology* 103, no. 3 (1992): 1075–1095.

Ensminger, A. H., M. E. Ensminger, J. E. Kolande, and J. R. Robson, eds. *Food and Nutrition Encyclopedia*, 2nd ed. Boca Raton, Fla.: CRC Press, 1994.

Filer, L. J., S. Garattini, M. R. Kare, W. A. Reynolds, and R. J. Wurtman. *Glutamic Acid: Advances in Biochemistry and Physiology*. New York: Raven Press, 1979.

Finn, R. "Food Allergy—Fact or Fiction: A Review." *Journal of the Royal Society of Medicine* 85, no. 9 (1992): 560–564.

Frieder, B., and V. E. Grim. "Prenatal Monosodium Glutamate (MSG) Treatment Given Through the Mother's Diet Causes Behavioral Deficits in Rat Offspring." *International Journal of Neuroscience* 23, no. 2 (1984): 117–126.

Gall, H., K. J. Kalveram, G. Forck, and W. Sterry. "Kiwi Fruit Allergy: A Newbirch Pollen Associated Food Allergy." *Journal of Allergy and Clinical Immunology* 94, no. 1 (1994): 70–76.

Goggins, M., and D. Kelleher. "Celiac Disease and Other Nutrient Related Injuries to the Gastrointestinal Tract." *American Journal of Gastrenterology* 89, no. 8 supplement (1994): S2–S17.

Golbert, T. M. "Food Allergy and Immunologic Diseases of the Gastrointestinal Tract." In *Allergic Diseases: Diagnosis and Management*, edited by R. Patterson. Philadelphia: J. B. Lippincott, 1993.

Hoffman, K. M., and H. A. Sampson. "Evaluation and Management of Patients with Adverse Food Reactions." In *Allergy, Asthma, and Immunology from Infancy to Adulthood*, edited by C. W. Bierman, D. S. Pearlman, G. G. Shapiro, and W. W. Busse. Philadelphia: W. B. Saunders, 1996.

Janatuinen, E. K., P. H. Pikkarainen, T. A. Kemppainen, V. M. Kosma, R. M. Jaarvinen, M. I. Uusitupa, and R. J. Julkunen. "A Comparison of Diets with and without Oats in Adults with Celiac Disease." *New England Journal of Medicine* 333, no. 16 (1995): 1033–1037.

Kelso, J. M., R. T. Jones, and J. W. Yuninger. "Oral Allergy Syndrome Successfully Treated with Pollen Immunotherapy." *Annals of Allergy, Asthma, and Immunology* 74, no. 5 (1995): 391–396.

Kemp, S. F., R. F. Lockey, B. L. Wolf, and P. Lieberman. "Anaphylaxis: A Review of 266 Cases." *Archives of Internal Medicine* 155, no. 16 (1995): 1749–1754.

Institute of Food Technologists' Expert Panel on Food Safety and Nutrition. "Monosodium Glutamate." *Food Technology* 41, no. 5 (1987): 143–145.

Lieberman, P., and J. A. Anderson, eds. *Allergic Diseases: Diagnosis and Treatment.* Totowa, N. J.: Humana Press, 1996.

Majamaa, H., P. Moisio, and K. Holm. "Cow's Milk Allergy: Diagnostic Accuracy of Skin Prick and Patch Tests and Specific IgE." *Allergy* 54 (1999): 346–351.

Malnick, S. D., Y. Lurie, M. Beergabel, and D. D. Bass. "Celiac Disease." *Postgraduate Medicine* 101, no. 6 (1997): 239–44.

Olney, J. W., O. L. Ho, and V. Rhee. "Brain Damaging Potentials of Protein Hydrolysates." *New England Journal of Medicine* 289, no. 8 (1973): 391–393.

Ortaloni, C., M. Ispano, E. A. Pastorello, R. Ansaloni, and G. C. Margi. "Comparison of Results of Skin Prick Tests (with Fresh Food and Commercial Food Extracts) and RAST in 100 Patients with Oral Allergy Syndrome." *Journal of Allergy and Clinical Immunology* 83, no. 3 (1989): 683–690.

Platts-Mills, T. A. "How the Environment Affects Children with Allergic Disease: Indoor Allergens and Asthma." *Annals of Allergy* 72, no. 4 (1994): 381–384.

Rasanen, L., M. Letho, K. Turjanman, J. Savolainen, and T. Reunala. "Allergy to Ingested Cereals in Atopic Children." *Allergy* 49, no. 10 (1994): 871–876.

Rostami, K., C. J. Mulder, J. M. Werre, F. R. van Beukelen, J. Kerchhaert, J. B. Crusius, A. S. Pena, F. L. Willekens, and J. W. Meijer. "High Prevalence of Celiac Disease in Apparently Healthy Blood Donors Suggests a High Prevalence of Undiagnosed Celiac Disease in the Dutch Population." *Scandinavian Journal of Gastroenterology* 34, no. 3 (1999): 276-9

Sampson, H. A., L. Medelson, and J. P. Rosen. "Fatal and Near-Fatal Anaphylactic Reactions to Foods in Children and Adolescents." *New England Journal of Medicine* 327, no. 6 (1992): 380–384.

Sampson, H. A. "Adverse Reactions to Foods." In *Allergy: Principles and Practice*, edited by E. Middleton, C. E. Reed, E. F. Ellis, N. F. Adkinson, J. W. Yunginger, and W. W. Busse. St. Louis: C. V. Mosby, 1993.

Shadick, N. A., M. H. Liang, A. J. Partridge, C. Bingham, E. Wright, A. H. Fossel, and A. L. Sheffer. "The Natural History of Exercise-Induced Anaphylaxis: Survey Results from a 10-Year Follow-up Study." *Journal of Allergy and Clinical Immunology* 104, no. 1 (1999): 123–127.

Souci, S. W., W. Fachmann, and H. Kraut, eds. *Food Composition and Nutrition Tables*. Stuttgart: Wissenschaftliche Verlegsgesellchaft, 1994.

Stegink, L. D., and L. J. Filer, eds. *Aspartame: Physiology and Biochemistry*. New York: Marcel Dekker, 1984.

Steinman, H. A. "Rostrum: 'Hidden' Allergens in Foods." *Journal of Allergy and Clinical Immunology* 98, no. 2 (1998): 241–250.

Tenaka, S. "An Epidemiological Survey on Food-Dependent Exercise-Induced Anaphylaxis in Kindergartners, Schoolchildren, and Junior High School Students." *Asia-Pacific Journal of Public Health* 7, no. 1 (1994): 26–30.

Tilles, S., A. Schocket, and H. Milgrom. "Exercise-Induced Anaphylaxis Related to Specific Foods." *Journal of Pediatrics* 127, no. 4 (1995): 587–589.

Unsworth, D. J., and D. L. Brown. "Serological Screening Suggests That Adult Celiac Disease Is Underdiagnosed in the U.K. and Increases the Incidence by up to 12%." *Gut* 35, no. 1 (1994): 61–64.

U.S. Food and Drug Administration. "FDA Backgrounder: FDA and Monosodium Glutamate (MSG)." (August 31, 1995). http://vm.cfsan.fda.gov/~lrd/msg.html (June 19, 1998).

Valenta, R., and D. Kraft. "Type 1 Allergic Reactions to Plant-Derived Food: A Consequence of Primary Sensitization to Pollen Allergens." *Journal of Allergy and Clinical Immunology* 97, no. 4 (1996): 893–895.

Winbourn, M. "Food Allergy, the Hidden Culprit." *Journal of American Academy of Nurse Practitioners* 6, no. 11 (1994): 515–522.

Wood, R. A. "Review of Environmental Control in the Prevention and Treatment of Pediatric Allergic Disease." *Current Opinion in Pediatrics* 5, no. 6 (1993): 692–695.

Yang, W. H., M. A. Drouin, M. Herbert, Y. Mao, and J. Karsh. "The Monosodium Glutamate Symptom Complex: Assessment in a Double-Blind, Placebo-Contolled, Randomized Study." *Journal of Allergy and Clinical Immunology* 99, no. 6 (1977): 757–762.

Yocum, M. W., and D. A. Khan. "Assessment of Patients Who Have Experienced Anaphylaxis: A 3-Year Survey." *Mayo Clinic Proceeding* 69, no. 1 (1994): 93.

INDEX

Page numbers in *italic* indicate recipes.